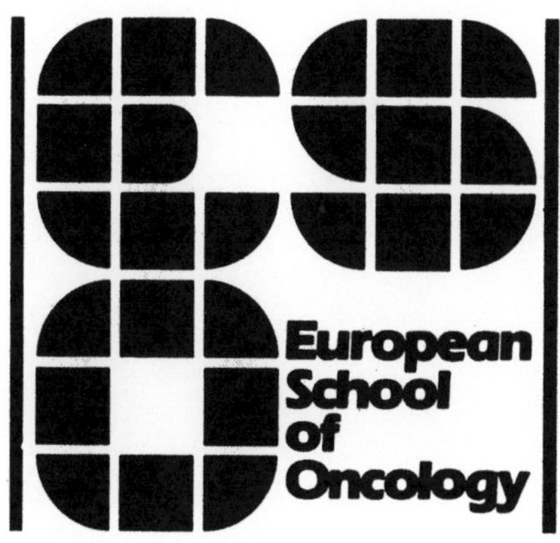

European
School
of
Oncology

AF307712

Monographs

Series Editor: U. Veronesi

R. Mertelsmann (Ed.)

Lymphohaematopoietic Growth Factors in Cancer Therapy

With 8 Figures and 14 Tables

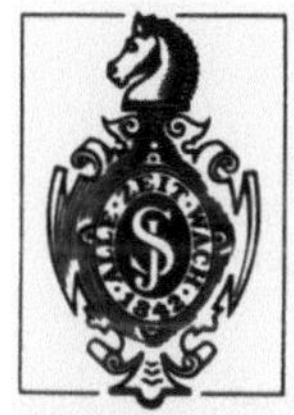

Springer-Verlag Berlin Heidelberg New York
London Paris Tokyo Hong Kong Barcelona

Abteilung Innere Medizin I
Klinikum der Albert-Ludwigs-Universität
Hugstetter Straße 55
7800 Freiburg
Federal Republic of Germany

The European School of Oncology gratefully acknowledges sponsorship for the Task Force received from ⟨Roche⟩ Prodotti Roche S.p.A. – Milano

Library of Concress Cataloging-in-Publication Data
Lymphohaematopoietic growth factors in cancer therapy / R. Mertelsmann (ed.). p. cm.– (Monographs / European School of Oncology)
ISBN-13: 978-3-642-76039-6   e-ISBN-13: 978-3-642-76037-2
DOI: 10.1007/ 978-3-642-76037-2
1. Cancer–Immunotherapy. 2. Hematopoietic growth factors–Therapeutic use. 3. Lymphokines–Therapeutic use. 4. Interleukins–Therapeutic use. I. Mertelsmann, Roland. II. Series: Monographs (European School of Oncology) [DNLM: 1. Growth Substances. 2. Interleukin-2–therapeutic use. 3. Interleukins–therapeutic use. 4. Killer Cells, Lymphokine-Activated. 5. Neoplasms–therapy. QZ 266 L9864] RC271.I45L944 1990 616.99'4061–dc20 DNLM/DLC for Library of Congress 90-10303 CIP

This work is subject to copyright. All rights are reserved, whether the whole or part of the material is concerned, specifically the rights of translation, reprinting, re-use of illustrations, recitation, broadcasting, reproduction on microfilms or in other ways, and storage in data banks. Duplication of this publication or parts thereof is only permitted under the provisions of the German Copyright Law of September 9, 1965, in its current version, and a copyright fee must always be paid. Violations fall under the prosecution act of the German Copyright Law.

© Springer-Verlag Berlin Heidelberg 1990
Softcover reprint of the hardcover 1st edition 1990

The use of general descriptive names, registered names, trademarks, etc. in this publication does not imply, even in the absence of a specific statement, that such names are exempt from the relevant protective laws and regulations and therefore free for general use.

Product Liability: The publisher can give no guarantee for information about drug dosage and application thereof contained in this book. In every individual case the respective user must check its accuracy by consulting other pharmaceutical literature.

2123/3145-543210 – Printed on acid-free paper

Foreword

The European School of Oncology came into existence to respond to a need for information, education and training in the field of the diagnosis and treatment of cancer. There are two main reasons why such an initiative was considered necessary. Firstly, the teaching of oncology requires a rigorously multidisciplinary approach which is difficult for the Universities to put into practice since their system is mainly disciplinary orientated. Secondly, the rate of technological development that impinges on the diagnosis and treatment of cancer has been so rapid that it is not an easy task for medical faculties to adapt their curricula flexibly.

With its residential courses for organ pathologies and the seminars on new techniques (laser, monoclonal antibodies, imaging techniques etc.) or on the principal therapeutic controversies (conservative or mutilating surgery, primary or adjuvant chemotherapy, radiotherapy alone or integrated), it is the ambition of the European School of Oncology to fill a cultural and scientific gap and, thereby, create a bridge between the University and Industry and between these two and daily medical practice.

One of the more recent initiatives of ESO has been the institution of permanent study groups, also called task forces, where a limited number of leading experts are invited to meet once a year with the aim of defining the state of the art and possibly reaching a consensus on future developments in specific fields of oncology.

The ESO Monograph series was designed with the specific purpose of disseminating the results of these study group meetings, and providing concise and updated reviews of the topic discussed.

It was decided to keep the layout relatively simple, in order to restrict the costs and make the monographs available in the shortest possible time, thus overcoming a common problem in medical literature: that of the material being outdated even before publication.

UMBERTO VERONESI
Chairman Scientific Committee
European School of Oncology

Contents

Introduction

Roland Mertelsmann

Department of Medicine I, Division of Haematology/Oncology, Albert-Ludwig's University Medical Centre, Hugstetter Strasse 55, 7800 Freiburg, FRG

Proliferation, differentiation and functional activity of haematopoietic and immunological progenitor and effector cells are regulated by a family of peptide hormones called cytokines. Recent information suggests an important role for these mediators not only in the elimination of pathogenic organisms and cells but also in the pathogenesis of infectious and neoplastic disorders. Studies of gene structure, gene expression, induction requirements and cellular sources using molecular probes and biological assays, have demonstrated a complex cascade of synergising activation signals that amplify immune and inflammatory responses. Through recombinant DNA technology, sufficient quantities of highly purified cytokines have become available for clinical evaluation.

Conceptually, cytokine-based treatment strategies are directed towards 1) stimulation of host antitumour defense mechanisms, 2) direct effect on tumour cell proliferation and differentiation, and 3) increasing host resistance to neoplasia- or therapy-induced lympho- and myelosuppression.

Interleukin 2 is the prime example of a cytokine which induces host effector cells with tumour killing capacities, resulting in reproducible albeit rare remissions in malignant melanoma and renal cell carcinoma. The interferons are thought to exert their most prominent clinical benefits in hairy cell leukaemia and chronic myelogenous leukaemia by direct effects on the respective leukaemic cell populations. Major progress has recently been made by using haematopoietic growth factors (haemopoietins) including erythropoietin, G-CSF, GM-CSF and Interleukin 3 in ameliorating disease- and therapy-induced myelosuppression with significant clinical benefits for patients. A survival advantage for patients receiving haemopoietins in conjunction with chemo/radiotherapy has already been demonstrated in some studies. A significant improvement in the quality of life of patients receiving cancer chemotherapy has been documented in all clinical studies so far, making the introduction of cytokines into the clinic one of the major advances in cancer therapy of the 1980s.

In preparing this monograph, the editor has had the privilege and pleasure to collaborate with an outstanding group of experts in clinical and experimental cytokine research, for which he expresses his warmest appreciation.

Interleukins and Haematopoietic Growth Factors

F.M. Rosenthal, A. Lindemann, F. Herrmann and R. Mertelsmann

Department of Medicine I, Division of Haematology/Oncology, Albert-Ludwig's University Medical Centre, Hugstetter Strasse 55, 7800 Freiburg, FRG

One of the most challenging areas of contemporary oncological and immunological research is represented by investigation of the potential clinical use of human cytokines.

In recent years, a breakthrough was provided by cloning of the genes of some of these growth factors. It was thus made possible to obtain homogeneous preparations of individual factors in sufficient quantities to permit large-scale laboratory and clinical trials.

For many years, standard treatment of malignant disease has focussed on local surgery, radiation and systemic chemotherapy. As the available therapy for the more frequent cancers has remained unsatisfactory, oncologists are forced to explore novel therapeutic approaches.

Improved understanding of tumour pathophysiology and immunology raises the possibility of introducing additional treatment modalities: the stimulation of host defense mechanisms including specific and non-specific immunological approaches as well as effects to directly affect tumour growth and differentiation by therapeutically influencing pathophysiological mechanisms. The complexity of the immune response to tumours necessitates a multifaceted approach to the problem of immunotherapy. Ideally, such an approach should attempt to minimise the ability of a tumour to escape immunological control, reduce tumour viability and enhance specific or non-specific host resistance. In practice, this may be achieved either by active manipulation of the immune response by vaccination against tumours or by administration of immunoregulatory factors such as cytokines. Another possible access to this problem is by passive immunotherapy involving the transfer of antibodies to cancer patients or by depletive immunotherapy, and finally by adoptive immunotherapy, entailing the transfer of immunocompetent cells from one individual to another or the administration of *ex vivo* activated autologous immune cells.

In this chapter, we will concentrate on the experience that has been gained with the use of cytokines in cancer therapy.

Cytokines are polypeptide products of activated cells which, in most instances, provide relatively short-range communication between a wide variety of cells by influencing their proliferation, differentiation and state of activation. They are produced by multiple cell types and several of them have pleiotropic and overlapping, sometimes synergistic or additive, activities that are not restricted to influencing one cell lineage only. The majority of growth factors appear to have the capacity of inducing other cytokines, including HGFs, in activated white blood cells. This complex network of interactions renders the evaluation of clinical studies conducted with these factors very complex, since multifaceted direct and indirect effects on many organ systems have to be expected.

The potential clinical use of human cytokines can arbitrarily be ramified into 4 strategies:

1. Stimulation of the immune response in order to enhance immunosurveillance of neoplasms (e.g., IL2).
2. Mitigation of cancer therapy and cancer-related immuno- and myelosuppression and augmentation of non-specific mechanisms of host resistance. (e.g., GM-CSF, G-CSF, EPO).
3. Indirect improvement of antitumour response and survival by reducing toxicity and thus altering the definition of the

Table 1. Cytokines involved in immunoregulation and haematopoietic blood cell development

Family	Molecules	Synonyms	Chromosomal localisation	Molecular weight* (kilodalton)
1. *Growth factors*	Multi-CSF	IL-3	5q23-q31	14-28
	GM-CSF	CSF-alpha	5q21-q32	14-35
	G-CSF	CSF-beta	17q11-q22	18-22
	M-CSF	CSF-1	5q33	47-74
	EPO		7q11-q22	34-39
2. *Interleukins*	IL-1	Hematopoietin-1	2q14	31;17
	IL-2	TCGF	4q26-q28	15.5
	IL-3	Multi-CSF	5q23-q31	14-28
	IL-4	BSF-1	5q	15-20
	IL-5	BCGF-II, TRF	5q	12-18
	IL-6	BSF-2	7q	24
3. *Interferons*	IFN-alpha	Leukocyte-IFN	9	18-20
	IFN-beta	Fibroblast-IFN	9	23
	IFN-gamma	Immune-IFN	12	20-25
4. *Tumor necrosis factors*	TNF-alpha	Cachectin	6	17
	TNF-beta	Lymphotoxin	6	25
5. *Others (examples)*	PDGF			
	TGF-alpha			
	TGF-beta			

TCGF, T-cell growth factor; BSF, B-cell stimulatory factor; BCGF, B-cell growth factor; TRF, T-cell replacing factor;
PDGF, platelet-derived growth factor; TGF, transforming growth factor
For other abbreviations see text
* Variations in molecular weight are in most cases due to different degrees of glycosylation

maximum tolerated doses of conventional chemotherapeutic regimens (CSFs).

4. Direct influence on tumour cell growth and differentiation via cytotoxic, cytostatic or regulatory mechanisms (e.g., TNF).

Apart from this potential use in cancer therapy, there are a number of non-neoplastic disorders associated with neutropenia, where the application of growth factors may prove to be beneficial.

Cytokines involved in immunoregulation or cell proliferation can be divided into several groups (Table 1), such as haematopoietic growth factors, interleukins, interferons, tumour necrosis factors, and others.

Since most cytokines possess pleiotropic biological properties, there are overlapping activities between groups, which makes any classification somewhat arbitrary.

Haematopoietic Growth Factors

The haematopoietic growth factors (HGFs) are a family of glycoprotein hormones which regulate survival, proliferation and differentiation of haematopoietic progenitor cells as well as the functional activities of mature cells [1] (see Fig. 1). During the past few years, the genes for 5 of the human factors have been defined and cloned, and recombinant forms of the proteins have been produced and purified. The different factors have been operationally defined by prefixes based on the predominant type of colony found *in vitro* in response to these molecules. The factors currently under active clinical investigation include multipotential colony-stimulating factor (Multi-CSF or interleukin 3), granulocyte-macrophage CSF (GM-CSF), granulocyte

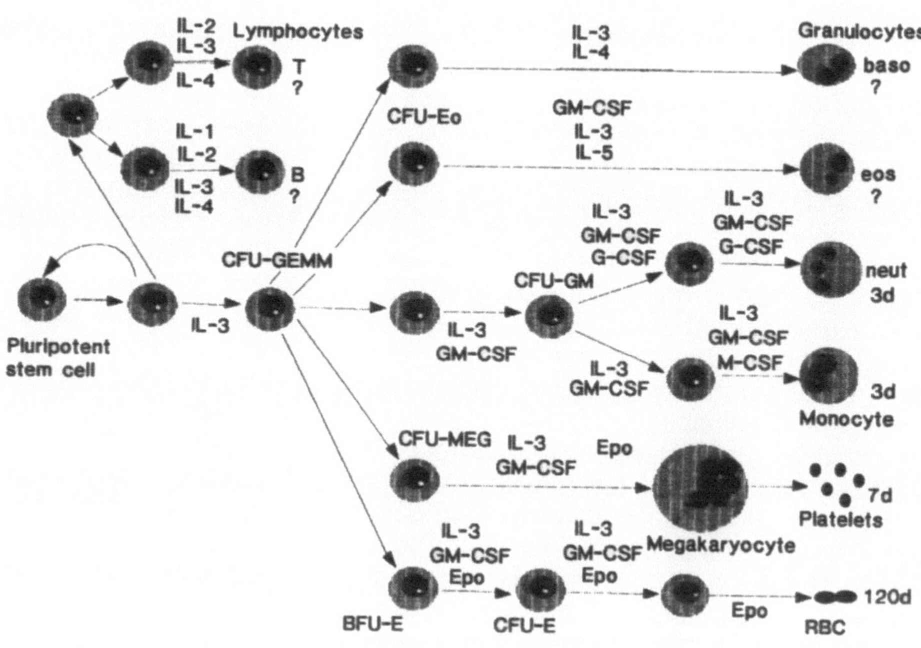

Fig. 1. Influence of haematopoietic growth factors on different cell types

CSF (G-CSF), macrophage CSF (M-CSF), and erythropoietin (EPO).

Granulocyte-Macrophage Colony-Stimulating Factor

The human gene encoding GM-CSF is located on chromosome 5q21-5q32 [2]. Probably due to variable glycolysation, the molecular mass of the mature protein, which comprises 127 amino acids, ranges from 14-35 kD [3]. A variety of cells producing GM-CSF have been identified, among them monocytes, fibroblasts, endothelial cells, epithelial cells and T lymphocytes [4]. GM-CSF stimulates granulocyte/macrophage and eosinophil colony formation *in vitro* and acts in combination with erythropoietin as erythroid burst promoting activity [5]. In addition to its effect on progenitor cell differentiation, GM-CSF also induces a variety of functional changes in mature cells. It increases neutrophil phagocytic activity, inhibits the migration of neutrophil granulocytes [6] and induces the production of other cytokines (e.g., TNF, IL1) by these same cells [7,8]. It also induces macrophage tumour cytotoxicity [9], activates macrophages to synthesise MHC class II molecules, to augment antigen pre-

sentation [10] and to release oxygen radicals [11].

Although these *in vitro* findings suggested a possible role for inducing indirect and direct antitumour effects, no such effects of GM-CSF could be observed in any of the clinical studies [12-14]. Induction of *in vivo* tumour cytotoxicity might be achieved by combining GM-CSF with more traditional macrophage activating factors like interferon-gamma (IFN-γ): GM-CSF delivering large numbers of effector cells and IFN-γ triggering the response.

Apart from its possible role as an antitumour agent, which requires further evaluation, GM-CSF demonstrates an already well characterised activity in reducing chemotherapy-associated morbidity.

Severe and prolonged myelosuppression after chemotherapy in neoplastic disease represents a fundamental problem. Complications during this myelosuppressive period often limit the practicability of chemotherapeutic regimens. Frequently, patients receiving high-dose chemotherapy develop neutropenia that often results in bacterial and secondary fungal infections. Shortening the period and degree of neutropenia should decrease the incidence and severity of infections and thereby also shorten hospital stay and even reduce mortality associated with chemotherapy.

In our own phase II clinical trial, it was shown that the neutrophil nadir was significantly elevated and time of relevant neutropenia was abbreviated with a single daily subcutaneous dose of GM-CSF (250 µg/m^2 body surface area) given over a period of 10 days [15]. Patients were protected from febrile events and incidence of mucositis was reduced as well. No significant effect was seen regarding platelet counts, haemoglobin levels or duration of chemotherapy-related thrombocytopenia and anaemia.

The toxicity encountered was tolerable. The adverse effects consisted mainly of discrete bone pain, skin rash and weakness. Short-lived dyspnoea was occasionally seen in patients receiving the factor intravenously, especially if white blood cell counts exceeded normal values by far. Dose-limiting toxicities reported were serositis and thrombosis with pulmonary emboli [16-21].

Effects of GM-CSF were also studied in the clinical setting of autologous bone marrow transplantation [17,22,23]. It has been shown that this growth factor increases the circulating pool of peripheral blood haematopoietic progenitors and thus accelerates the rate of neutrophil recovery. No difference was seen with respect to the first appearance of neutrophils in the circulation when comparing GM-CSF-treated patients with non-treated patients [24]. This may open new perspectives in the field of bone marrow transplantation. The need for bone marrow harvesting might be avoided by using peripheral blood stem cells for transplantation.

Application of GM-CSF to patients with myelodysplastic syndrome (MDS) has been described to normalise red-cell, white-cell and platelet counts in some patients [25]. More recent studies, however, have not been able to confirm this optimistic report, demonstrating rises in neutrophil counts only. At higher GM-CSF doses, an increase in leukaemic blast cells in the bone marrow was seen, indicating that GM-CSF can stimulate the proliferation of human leukaemic blast cells as well as normal haematopoietic cells *in vivo* [19,20,26]. Even a possible progression to frank leukaemia has been observed [26]. On the other hand, in the future one might be able to take advantage of blastoge-nesis induced *in vivo*, by augmenting the proportion of malignant cells recruited into the S-phase of the cell cycle and thus obtain enhanced cytotoxic effects with drugs such as Ara-C, that kill cycle-activated cells [27,28].

The value of GM-CSF in the treatment of aplastic anaemia appears to be limited, as reported by Champlin and Nissen [29,30]. Combinations of haematopoietic growth factors acting on early progenitors with later-acting factors might have synergistic effects in accelerating repopulation of the bone marrow and warrant further investigation in this disease.

Ultimately, GM-CSF may find a place in the treatment of other non-malignant conditions which are characterised by leukopenia (e.g., AIDS) [31], or in the improvement of host defence in infectious disease complications [32].

Granulocyte Colony-Stimulating Factor

By recombinant DNA technology, 2 cDNAs representing a 177 amino-acid protein form and a 174 amino-acid protein form of human granulocyte colony-stimulating factor (G-CSF) could be isolated [33-35]. It is not known, however, whether both forms do physiologically exist in man. The shorter version of the molecules seems to be more active *in vivo*. The gene which encodes for G-CSF is located on chromosome 17 in region q11-q22 [36].

G-CSF is a rather lineage-specific haematopoietic growth factor in that it acts on cells capable of forming one differentiated cell type: the neutrophil granulocyte. In combination with other haematopoietic growth factors, it acts synergistically to stimulate a broader spectrum of colony-forming units [33]. In addition, G-CSF increases antibody-dependent cellular cytotoxicity of peripheral blood granulocytes as well as several other aspects of neutrophil activity [37].

Like GM-CSF, G-CSF has been utilised in the prevention of chemotherapy-induced neutropenia [38-42] and in the setting of autologous bone marrow transplantation [22,43]. A dose-dependent increase in absolute neutrophil counts (at least 3-fold) and shortening of the neutropenic period was observed. At higher doses, an up to 10-fold increase in monocytes was also seen [40]. In one study, the incidence of severe infections was reduced following those cycles of chemotherapy combined with G-CSF [39].

Neutropenia caused by marrow infiltration with low-grade lymphoma (hairy-cell leukaemia) also improved after treatment with G-CSF [44].

Toxicities in G-CSF trials in general have been minimal, essentially being limited to bone pain, presumably secondary to bone marrow expansion. This adverse effect was seen in up to 25% of patients treated with an intravenous bolus of $\geq$30 µg/kg of body weight; with subcutaneous administration and lower doses it was encountered less frequently. In some patients, reversible elevation of serum alkaline phosphatase and lactic dehydrogenase has been noted and, occasionally, evidence of overshooting neutrophil activation such as acute neutrophilic dermatosis (Sweet's Syndrome) has been observed [44]. Preliminary data from an ongoing phase III study in the USA show a reduction of platelet counts after repeated subcutaneous injections of G-CSF (240 µg/m^2/day for 14 days of repeated 21-day chemotherapy cycles). Whether this clinical result can only be ascribed to G-CSF has not been clarified yet.

Again, like GM-CSF, G-CSF is currently being tested by a number of investigators for its usefulness in the treatment of neutropenic disorders not due to malignancies, e.g., congenital (Kostmann's Syndrome), cyclic or idiopathic neutropenia [45-47]. From the promising preliminary data it can be anticipated that, in the near future, some of these disorders can be at least ameliorated by the application of recombinant G-CSF.

Erythropoietin

Erythropoietin (EPO) is a glycoprotein hormone, produced predominantly in the kidney and to a small extent in the liver. It regulates proliferation and differentiation of erythroid progenitor cells to mature erythrocytes [48]. Recent work has suggested that the EPO-producing cell in the kidney is a peritubular interstitial cell found mainly in the inner renal cortex [49,50]. In the adult, only 10-20% of plasma-EPO are produced in the liver but the exact site of synthesis has not been identified yet [51]. In the foetus, however, the liver is the primary site of EPO formation [52].

The mechanism by which a hypoxic stimulus triggers the production and release of EPO is still unknown. Evidence has been presented that the oxygen sensor is a haeme protein [53].

EPO is a heavily glycosylated, 166 amino acids containing protein with a molecular mass of 34-39 kD. The EPO gene has been localised to chromosome 7q11-q22 by *in-situ* hybridisation [54]. Like for its natural counterpart, the major target cells for recombinant EPO have been identified as colony-forming progenitor cells committed to the erythroid lineage (CFU-E, colony forming unit-erythroid) and, to a lesser extent, more immature erythroid progenitor cells: the BFU-E (burst forming unit-erythroid). Although some *in-vivo* data have been accumulated indicating that EPO induces the proliferation of megakaryocyte (CFU-MK) and granulocyte/macrophage (CFU-GM) progenitor cells [55-57], in most of the recent clinical trials no significant changes in circulating leukocyte or platelet numbers were seen. This, however, may be related to dose and time schedule of EPO administration in these studies.

Clinical studies have clearly documented the effectiveness of recombinant EPO in correction of anaemia in patients with end-stage renal disease [58,59] as well as in pre-dialysis patients [60]. In these patients, only low levels of EPO can be demonstrated in the serum. Although, pathogenetically, anaemia in tumour patients is not characterised by EPO-deficiency, we investigated whether EPO-levels exceeding normal values could stimulate erythropoiesis in these patients and thus contribute to correcting transfusion-dependent anaemia.

The therapeutic effect of EPO in correcting chemotherapy-induced anaemia in patients with normal renal function was demonstrated recently [61]. A significant and sustained increase in haemoglobin and haematocrit was demonstrated with EPO given twice weekly as a bolus injection at an escalating dose schedule (150-300 U/kg body weight). EPO response was accompanied by changes of ferrokinetics, as measured by serum ferritin which was significantly reduced by the end of therapy. The requirement for red blood cell transfusion was eliminated by EPO therapy.

EPO was also shown to be beneficial in the treatment of anaemia of malignancy due to neoplastic bone marrow infiltration [62]. One patient with multiple myeloma showed an increase of platelet counts by >75% above the baseline level, which was maintained for some time (2-3 months) after EPO discontinuation. This result underlines that the potential role of EPO as a thrombopoietic growth factor needs further evaluation.

No side effects were noted during EPO-therapy. This conflicts with results in patients with end-stage renal disease, where EPO-therapy was associated with increases in blood pressure and where even thromboses, strokes and seizures, induced by increases in peripheral vascular resistance and blood viscosity, were seen. This difference can possibly be explained by a predisposition of patients with renal disease to vascular complications.

Interleukin 3 (Multi-CSF)

Like for GM- and G-CSF, the gene for Interleukin 3 (IL3) has been located on the long arm of chromosome 5 in region q23-q31 [63]. The protein is produced by activated T lymphocytes and has a molecular mass of 14-28 kD. IL3 is a multi-lineage haematopoietin which promotes the growth and differentiation of various myeloid progenitor cells including early multipotent progenitors such as blast colony-forming units and mixed colonies. The colonies produced in response to IL3 contain eosinophils, basophils, neutrophils, mast cells, megacaryocytes, macrophages and erythroid cells.

In preclinical murine and primate models, IL3 has been shown to significantly elevate numbers of circulating leukocytes [64,65]. A phase I/II trial in patients with advanced malignancies with or without bone marrow failure has revealed the following dose-related haematological responses: increases in platelet counts, absolute leukocyte counts, reticulocyte counts and bone marrow cellularity [66]. Side effects included fever, flushing, headache and local irritation at the site of injection. More efficacy is to be expected by using combinations of haematopoietins acting on early progenitor cells with late-acting myeloid growth factors.

Macrophage Colony-Stimulating Factor

Macrophage colony-stimulating factor (M-CSF) is the last of the human haematopoietic growth factors available in recombinant form which has just progressed from the laboratory into clinical use. Definite data with respect to biological activity and toxicity in man are not yet available.

M-CSF is a glycoprotein of 47-74 kD comprising two identical subunits [67]. The gene is located on chromosome 5 in close proximity to the IL3 gene (5q33). Monocytes, fibroblasts and endothelial cells are producers of this factors.

Interleukins

Of all interleukins known to affect the immune response, Interleukin 2 (IL2) has received most attention in cancer therapy.

IL2, previously known as T-cell growth factor, is a 15.5 kD glycoprotein secreted predominantly by T-helper lymphocytes after exposure to mitogens or antigens. It induces T-cell proliferation and the proliferation and differentiation of B-cells, resulting in the secondary induction of other lymphokines, including IL4 [68], Tumour Necrosis Factor (TNF) [69] and IFN-γ [70,71]. IFN-γ, in turn, is the prototype of a macrophage-activating factor enhancing, for example, the ability of macrophages to kill intracellular pathogens and tumour cells [72-75].

IL2 also directly augments the cytotoxicity of human monocytes [76] and stimulates the activation of non-specific cytolytic effector cells designated lymphokine-activated killer (LAK) cells.

Most of the IL2-induced cytolytic activity was found to be mediated by NK cells [77].

Experiments with sublethally irradiated tumour-bearing animals suggested that recombinant IL2 does not cause tumour regression by a direct action on the tumour but rather by activation of a radiosensitive host component, presumably some cellular component of the immune system [78]. The potential clinical use of IL2 thus depends on its ability to activate endogenous or exogenous cells able to exert antitumour effects.

Initial clinical studies with IL2 were performed by Rosenberg and colleagues, who used adoptive immunotherapy with high-dose IL2 and *ex vivo* activated LAK cells in patients with metastatic malignant melanoma (MM), renal cell carcinoma (RCC) or colorectal cancer [79,80]. This protocol consists of an i.v. IL2 bolus injection of 10^4-10^5 U/kg body weight every 8 hours for 5 days to stimulate LAK precursor cells, followed by the harvest of peripheral blood lymphocytes by leukapheresis and subsequent *in-vitro* cultivation and stimulation with IL2. These LAK cells are then reinfused into the patient with an additional systemic bolus dose of IL2. West and colleagues described a continuous infusion regimen for IL2 plus LAK cells which produced comparable results with apparently lower toxicity [81].

Antitumour activity could also be demonstrated in patients with MM or RCC receiving IL2 therapy without LAK cells, indicating that exogenous LAK cells are not an absolute requirement for antitumour activity of IL2.

Overall response rates achieved by IL2 treatment with or without LAK cells ranged from 0-50% in RCC and 11-50% in MM [80,82-84].

Side effects of IL2 were significant in patients treated on high-dose protocols. The dose-limiting toxicities included fever and chills, hypotension and interstitial pulmonary oedema, due to the development of a capillary leak syndrome. These effects were resolved within 24-48 hours after discontinuation of therapy. Other commonly encountered side effects were nausea/vomiting, diarrhoea and bone marrow toxicity (anaemia, thrombocytopenia). In the pathogenesis of adverse events, IL2-induced release of prostaglandins and other secondary mediators like TNF-alpha or IL1 are thought to play a role [85-87].

An interesting phenomenon that is frequently reported and also observed in our ongoing study with IL2 plus IFN-alpha (repeated cycles of a 96-hour infusion of IL2 in a dose of 3 MU/m^2/day and subcutaneous injection of IFN-alpha in a dose of 6 MU/m^2/day on day 1 and 4) in patients with MM and RCC is mixed responses, suggesting a different susceptibility of metastases to treatment depending on their anatomical site. Preliminary results of

this trial show comparable efficacy (response rate of 24%) to the trial using IL2 and LAK cells with reduced toxicity (unpublished observation).

To investigate the possible synergistic effects of IL2 with chemotherapeutic agents, clinical studies using IL2 in conjunction with low-dose cyclophosphamide in patients with MM and RCC have been conducted [88-90]. The rationale for adding this cytotoxic drug was to block induction of counteracting suppressor T lymphocytes by IL2. In the clinical trials, no objective responses were achieved in patients with RCC, and 15-43% remission rates (complete and partial remissions and mixed responses) were seen in melanoma patients. Responses to IL2 alone or in combination with LAK cells or cyclophosphamide have been seen with a variety of doses and schedules, but at the present time no optimal regimen can be defined.

Another immuotherapeutic approach to the treatment of patients with malignant melanoma was reported by Rosenberg [91]. With the systemic administration of *ex vivo* expanded tumour-infiltrating lymphocytes (TIL) in conjunction with IL2 and pretreatment of patients with cyclophosphamide, apparently higher response rates were achieved in a preliminary clinical trial than with the treatment with LAK cells. Duration of response, however, was often short.

Tumour Necrosis Factor Alpha

Tumour Necrosis Factor alpha (TNF-alpha), a secretory product of activated macrophages [69,92,93], NK cells, T lymphocytes, B lymphocytes and also granulocytes [94,95], is an endogenous mediator of inflammation and various immunological reactions. The protein has a molecular weight of 17 kD and is encoded by a gene located on the short arm of chromosome 6 [96,97]. It has been shown that TNF can activate neutrophils [98], augment macrophage [99] and NK cell [100] cytotoxicity and induce other cytokines such as IL1 and IL6 [101]. *In vitro* experiments have also demonstrated several effects of TNF on vascular endothelium, e.g., induction of MHC antigens [102], increased adherence for granulocytes [103], inhibition of endothelial growth [104] and also, paradoxically, stimulation of angiogenesis [105].

The ability of TNF to show cytotoxic activity for many transformed cell lines but not normal cells [106] and its antitumour activity in animal models [107,108], led to its clinical evaluation in cancer patients: in phase I and II studies with single-agent TNF, the overall response rate was disappointingly low, ranging around 5%, and toxicity was substantial. Slightly higher response rates were seen in gastrointestinal tumours and RCC [109,110].

At lower doses, general weakness, fever and chills dominated the clinical picture. As reported for IL2, the dose-limiting toxicity was hypotension and interstitial fluid retention. Other, also mainly dose-dependent adverse effects, were nausea/vomiting, diarrhoea, headache and myalgia [110]. The most frequently observed laboratory abnormality was a temporary decrease in absolute leukocyte counts. This is most likely due to redistribution or margination of circulating leukocytes by TNF-induced increased endothelial adherence [111,112].

The effects by which TNF exerts its antitumour activity are pleiotropic and not yet understood. Evidence has been presented that direct and indirect vascular effects via activation of the arachidonic acid cascade are involved in the induction of tumour necrosis and also in TNF-induced side effects. Animal experiments have shown that the administration of oxygen scavengers could prevent lethality without impairment of the antitumour activity [113]. It remains to be seen, in clinical trials, whether pretreatment with oxygen scavengers or the combination of TNF with other immunoregulatory agents reduces side effects without inhibiting antitumour effects.

Interferons

Interferons (IFNs) are a heterogeneous family of proteins which have been broadly classified into 3 groups: alpha, beta and gamma. IFN-alpha and IFN-beta ("type I IFNs") have similar biological and physico-chemical properties and are produced following viral infections by leukocytes and fibroblasts, respectively. IFN-gamma or immune IFN ("type II IFN") is secreted by antigen- or mitogen-activated T lymphocytes. The properties attributed to the various IFNs are numerous and include antiviral activity, antiproliferative and immunomodulatory effects. The antineoplastic activity would seem to result from both a direct inhibitory effect on cell growth and multiplication [114] and an indirect effect by modification of the immune system. The latter effect includes augmentation of NK-cell activity [115], increased expression of surface antigens [116] and suppression or enhancement of some B- and T-cell functions [117,118]. IFN-gamma is also a potent activator of macrophage function [75,119].

Up to now, the most impressive clinical results have been achieved with IFN-alpha in haematological disorders, especially in hairy-cell leukaemia [120] and chronic myelogenous leukaemia [121]. IFN-alpha has also been recommended for the treatment of AIDS-related Kaposi's sarcoma [122] and malignant melanoma [123].

Clinical trials with IFN-alpha in patients with hairy-cell leukaemia (HCL) have shown remission rates between 70-90%, with 10-30% complete remissions (CR) [124]. After cessation of treatment, up to 40% of CRs relapsed within 9-12 months. However, remissions could be easily reinduced in these patients when IFN-alpha therapy was resumed [125]. The mechanism by which IFN-alpha acts in HCL is uncertain. There is evidence that exogenous IFN-alpha may interrupt an endocrine loop in which responder cells other than hairy cells produce cytokines (e.g., TNF) that inhibit normal haematopoiesis and stimulate the growth of hairy cells [126,127].

Chronic myelogenous leukaemia (CML) is also sensitive to IFN-alpha. Recently, Talpaz described a 73% complete haematological remission rate in 96 patients with early benign phase CML [128]. Nineteen percent of the patients achieved a cytogenetic remission with a complete suppression of the clone carrying the Philadelphia chromosome. Of the responding patients, 60% have sustained complete cytogenetic responses for >6 months, the median duration being 30 months.

Also patients who relapse with CML after allogenic bone marrow transplantation might benefit from IFN-alpha therapy [129].

The results in late chronic phase (time from diagnosis >1 year) have been less favourable. Here, a possible approach might be a combination treatment of IFN-alpha and low-dose cytosine arabinoside [130].

Adverse events observed with IFN therapy are predominantly flu-like symptoms such as fever, chills, fatigue and myalgias. Anorexia, weight loss, nausea/vomiting and diarrhoea were also frequently reported.

The laboratory abnormalities seen during therapy with IFN indicated mild haematological (leukopenia, anaemia, neutropenia, thrombocytopenia), renal (proteinuria, elevated BUN) and hepatic (elevated GOT and bilirubin) toxicity [131].

Other indications in oncology for which IFN has proved promising, but in which it has not yet received widespread approval, include multiple myeloma [124], T-cell lymphoma [132] and non-Hodgkin's lymphoma [133] and RCC [134].

REFERENCES

1   Nicola NA: Why do hematopoietic growth factor receptors interact with each other? Immunol Today 1987 (8):134-139

2   Hueber K, Isobe M, Croce CM, Golde DM, Kaufman SE, Gasson JC: The human gene encoding GM-CSF is a 5q29-q32, the chromosome region deleted in the 5q-anomaly. Science 1985 (230):1282-1285

3   Donahue RE, Wang EA, Foutch L, Leary AC, Witek-Giametti JS, Metzger M, Hewick RM, Steinbrink DR, Shaw G: Effects of N-linked carbohydrate on the in vivo properties of human GM-CSF. Cold Spring Harbour Symp Quant Biol 1986 (51):685-692

4   Herrmann F, Oster W, Meuer SC, Klein K, Lindemannn A, Mertelsmann R: Interleukin-1 stimulates T lymphocytes to produce GM-CSF. J Clin Invest 1988 (81):1415-1418

5   Donahue RE, Emerson SG, Wang EA, Wong GG, Clark SC, Nathan DG: Demonstration of burst-promoting activity of recombinant human GM-CSF on circulating erythroid progenitors using an assay involving the delayed addition of erythropoietin. Blood 1985 (66):1479-1481

6   Metcalf D, Begley CG, Johnson GR, Nicola NA, Vadas MA, Lopez AF, Williamson DJ, Wong GG, Clark SC, Wang EA: Biologic properties in vitro of recombinant human granulocyte-macrophage colony-stimulating factor. Blood 1986 (67):37-45

7   Lindemann A, Riedel D, Oster W, Meuer SC, Blohm D, Mertelsmann R, Herrmann F: GM-CSF induces secretion of interleukin-1 by polymorphonuclear neutrophils. J Immunol 1988 (140):837-839

8   Herrmann F, Riedel D, Bambach T, Mertelsmann R: Recombinant granulocyte/macrophage-colony stimulating factor (RGM-CSF) inhibits growth of clonogenic cells in monoblast line U937 due to induction of tumor necrosis factor-alpha (TNF-ALPHA) and interleukin 1 (IL-1). Proc Am Soc Clin Oncol 1987 (6):A71

9   Grabstein KH, Urdal DL, Tushinsi RJ, Mochizuki DY, Price VL, Canterell MA, Gillis S, Conlon PJ: Induction of macrophage tumoricidal activity by GM-CSF. Science 1986 (32):506-508

10 Fischer H-G, Frosch S, Reske K, Reske-Kunz AB: GM-CSF activates macrophages derived from bone marrow cultures to synthesis of MHC class II molecules and to augmented antigen presentation function. J Immunol 1988 (141):3882-3888

11 Reed SG, Nathan CF, Pihl DL, Rodricks P, Shanebeck K, Conlon PJ, Grabstein PJ: Recombinant granulocyte/macrophage colony stimulating factor activates macrophages to inhibit Trypanosoma cruzi and release hydrogen peroxide: Comparison with y-interferon. J Exp Med 1987 (166):1734-1746

12 Herrmann F, Schulz G, Lindemann A, Meyenburg W, Oster W, Krumwieh D, Mertelsmann R: Yeast-expressed granulocyte-macrophage colony-stimulating factor in cancer patients: A phase Ib clinical study. Behring Inst Mitt 1988 (83):107-118

13 Steis RG, Clark J, Longo DL: A phase Ib evaluation of recombinant granulocyte-macrophage colony-stimulating factor. In: Berger HG et al (eds) Cancer Therapy. Springer-Verlag, Berlin, Heidelberg 1989 pp 103-111

14 Herrmann F, Schulz G, Lindemann A, Meyenburg W, Oster W, Krumwieh D, Mertelsmann R: Hematopoietic responses in patients with advanced malignancy treated with recombinant human granulocyte-macrophage colony-stimulating factor. J Clin Oncol 1989 (7):159-167

15 Herrmann F, Wieser M, Schulz G, Lindemann A, Oster W, Mertelsmann R: Single daily subcutaneous administration of rhGM-CSF ameliorates hematopoietic toxicity of chemotherapy in outpatinets. Blood 1988 (72): Abstr 390

16 Link H, Freund M, Kirchner H, Stoll M, Schmid H, Bucsky P, Seidel J, Schulz G, Schmidt RE, Riehm H, Poliwoda H, Welte K: Enhancement of autologous bone marrow transplantation with recombinant granulocyte-macrophage colony-stimulating factor (rhGM-CSF). In: Berger HG et al (eds) Cancer Therapy. Springer-Verlag, Berlin, Heidelberg 1989 pp 96-102

17 Brandt SJ, Peters WP, Atwater SK, Kurtzberg J, Borowitz MJ, Jones RB, Shpall EJ, Bast RC, Gilbert CJ, Oette DH: Effect of recombinant human granulocyte-macrophage colony-stimulating factor on hematopoietic reconstitution after high-dose chemotherapy and autologous bone marrow transplantation. N Engl J Med 1988 (318):869-876

18 Antman KS, Griffin JD, Elias A, Socinski MA, Ryan L, Cannistra SA, Oette D, Whitley M, Frei E, Schnipper LE: Effect of recombinant human granulocyte-macrophage colony-stimulating factor on chemotherapy-induced myelosuppression. N Engl J Med 1988 (319):593-598

19 Ganser A, Völkers B, Greher J, Ottmann OG, Walther F, Becker R, Bergmann L, Schulz G, Hoelzer D: Recombinant human granulocyte-macrophage colony-stimulating factor in patients with myelodysplastic syndromes - a phase I/II trial. Blood 1989 (73):31-37

20 Ganser A, Völkers B, Greher J, Walther F, Hoelzer D: Application of granulocyte-macrophage colony-stimulating factor in patients with malignant hematological diseases. In: Berger HG et al (eds) Cancer Therapy. Springer-Verlag, Berlin, Heidelberg 1989 pp 90-95

21 Herrmann F, Ganser A, Lindemann A, Wieser M, Schulz G, Hoelzer D, Mertelsmann R: Stimulation of granulopoiesis in patients with malignancy by rhGM-CSF: Assessment of two routes of administration. J Biol Response Mod 1989 (in press)

22 Peters WP: The effect of recombinant human colony-stimulating factors on hematopoietic reconstitution following autologous bone marrow transplantation. Sem Hematol 1989 (26):18-23

23 Peters WP, Atwater S, Kurtzberg J: The use of recombinant human granulocyte macrophage colony-stimulating factor in autologous bone marrow transplantation. In: Gale R, Champlin R (eds) Bone Marrow Transplantation: Current Controversies. A Liss, New York 1989 pp 595-606

24 Socinski MA, Cannistra SA, Elias A, Antman KH, Schnipper L, Griffin JD: Granulocyte-macrophage

colony stimulating factor expands the circulating hematopoietic progenitor cell compartment in man. Lancet 1988 (1):1194-1198

25 Vadhan-Raj S, Keating M, LeMaistre A, Hittelman WN, McCredie K, Trujillo JM, Broxmeyer HE, Henney C, Gutterman JU: Effects of recombinant human granulocyte-macrophage colony-stimulating factor in patients with myelodysplastic syndrome. N Engl J Med 1987 (317):1545-1552

26 Herrmann F, Lindemann A, Klein H, Luebbert M, Schulz G, Mertelsmann R: Effect of recombinant human granulocyte-macrophage colony-stimulating factor in patients with myelodysplastic syndrome with excess blasts. Leukemia 1989 (3):335-338

27 Cannistra SA, Groshek P, Griffin JD: Granulocyte-macrophage colony-stimulating factor enhances the cytotoxic effects of cytosine-arabinoside in acute myeloblastic leukemia and in the myéloid blast crisis phase of chronic myeloid leukemia. Leukemia 1989 (3):328-334

28 Andreeff M, Hegewisch-Becker S, Tafuri A, Bressler J, Redner A, Haimi J, Souza L, Welte K: Recruitment of leukemic cells in vitro by colony-stimulating factors (G-CSF, GM-CSF, Interleukin-3): evidence of increased cell kill and of differentiation by high-and low-dose cytosine arabinoside. Blut 1989 (in press)

29 Champlin RE, Nimer SD, Ireland P, Oette DH, Golde DW: Treatment of refractory aplastic anaemia with recombinant human granulocyte-macrophage colony-stimulating factor. Blood 1989 (73):694-699

30 Nissen C, Tichelli A, Gratwohl A, Speck B, Milne A, Gordon-Smith EC, Schaedelin J: Failure of recombinant human granulocyte-macrophage colony-stimulating factor therapy in aplastic anaemia patients with severe neutropenia. Blood 1988 (72):2045-2047

31 Groopman J, Mitsuyasu RT, DeLero M, Oette DH, Golde DW: Effect of recombinant human granulocyte-macrophage colony-stimulating factor on myelopoiesis in the acquired immmunodeficiency syndrome. N Engl J Med 1987 (317):593-598

32 Mooney DP, Ganelli RL, O'Reeilly M, Herbert JC: Recombinant human granulocyte colony-stimulating factor and pseudomonas burn wound sepsis. Arch Surg 1988 (123):1353-1357

33 Welte K, Platzer E, Lu L, Gabrilove JL, Levi E, Mertelsmann R, Moore MAS: Purification and biological characterization of human pluripotent hematopoietic colony-stimulating factor. Proc Natl Acad Sci USA 1985 (82):1526-1530

34 Nagata S, Tsuchiya M, Asano S, Kaziro Y, Yamazaki T, Yamamozo O, Hirata N, Kubota N, Oheda H, Nomura H, Ono M: Molecular cloning and expression of cDNA for human granulocyte colony-stimulating factor. Nature 1986 (319):415-418

35 Souza LM, Boone TC, Gabrilove JL, Lai PH, Zsebok M, Murdock DC, Chazin VR, Bruszewski J, Lu H, Chen KK, Barendt J, Platzer E, Moore MAS, Mertelsmann R, Welte K: Recombinant human granulocyte colony-stimulating factor: effects on normal and leukemic myeloid cells. Science 1986 (232):61-65

36 Simmers RN, Webber LM, Shannon MF, Garson OM, Wong MA, Sutherland GR: Localization of the G-CSF gene on chromosome 17 proximal to the breakpoint in the t(15;17) in acute promyelocytic leukemia. Blood 1987 (70):330-332

37 Platzer E, Oez K, Welte, K, Sandler A, Gabrilove JL, Mertelsman R, Moore MA, Kalden JR: Human pluripotent hematopoietic colony stimulating factor; activities on human and murine cells. Immunobiol 1987 (172):185-193

38 Asano S, Shirafuji N, Watari K, Matsuda S, Uemura N, Jeki R, Kodo H, Takaku F: Phase I clinical study for recombinant human granulocyte colony-stimulating factor. Behring Inst Mitt 1988 (83):222-228

39 Bronchud M, Scarfte JH, Thatcher N, Crowther D, Souza LM, Alton NK, Testa NG, Dexter TM: Phase I/II study of recombinant human granulocyte colony-stimulating factor in patients receiving intensive chemotherapy for small cell lung cancer. Br J Cancer 1987 (56):809-813

40 Gabrilove JL, Jakubowski A, Scher H, Sternberg C, Wong G, Gron J, Yagoda A, Fain K, Moore MAS, Clarkson B, Oettgen HF, Alton K, Welte K, Souza L: Effect of granulocyte colony-stimulating factor on neutropenia and associated morbidity due to chemotherapy or transitional cell carcinoma of the urothelium. N Engl J Med 1988 (318):1414-1422

41 Lindemann A, Herrmann F, Oster W, Meyenburg W, Haffneer P, Souza L, Mertelsmann R: Hematologic effects of recombinat human granulocyte colony-stimulating factor in patients with malignancy. Blood 1989 (in press)

42 Morstyn G, Campbell L, Souza LM, Alton NK, Keech J, Green M, Sheridan W, Metcalf D, Fox R: Effect of granulocyte colony-stimulating factor on neutropenia induced by cytotoxic chemotherapy. Lancet 1988 (1):667-672

43 Sheridan W, Morstyn G, Green M et al: Phase II study of granulocyte colony-stimulating factor (G-CSF) in autologous bone marrow transplantation (ABMT). Proc Am Soc Clin Oncol 1990 (abstr in press)

44 Glapsy JA, Baldwin GC, Robertson PA, Souza L, Vincent M, Ambersley J, Golde DW: Therapy for neutropenia in hairy cell leukemia with recombinant human granulocyte colony-stimulating factor. Ann Intern Med 1988 (109):789-795

45 Jakubowski AA, Souza L, Kelly F, Fain K, Budman D, Clarkson B, Bonilla MA, Moore MAS, Gabrilove J: Effects of granuolcyte colony-stimulating factor in a patient with idiopathic neutropenia. N Engl J Med 1989 (320):38-42

46 Hammond WP, Price TH, Souza LM, Dale DC: Treatment of cyclic neutropenia with granulocyte colony-stimulating factor. N Engl J Med 1989 (320):1306-1311

47 Bonilla MA, Gillio AP, Ruggiero M, Kernan NA, Brochstein JA, Abboud MA, Fumagalli L, Vincent M, Welte K, Souza LM, O'Reilly RI: In vivo recombinant human granulocyte colony-stimulating factor (rhG-CSF) corrects neutropenia in patients with congenital agranulocytosis: Blood 1988 (72):Abstr 349

48   Spivac JL: The mechanism of action of erythropoietin. Int J Cell Cloning 1986 (4):139-166

49   Koury ST, Bondurant MC, Koury MJ: Localization of erythropoietin synthesizing cells in murine kidneys by in situ hybridization. Blood 1988 (71):524-527

50   Lacombe C, DaSilva JL, Bruneval P, Fournier JG, Wendling F, Casadevall N, Camilleri JP, Bariety J, Varet B, Tambourin P: Peritubular cells are the site of erythropoietin synthesis in the murine hypoxic kidney. J Clin Invest 1988 (81):620-623

51   Fried W: The liver as a source of extrarenal erythropoietin production. Blood 1972 (40):671-677

52   Zanjani ED, Poster J, Burlington H, Mann LI, Wasserman LR: Liver as the primary site of erythropoietin formation in the fetus. J Lab Clin Med 1977 (89):640-644

53   Goldberg MA, Dunning SP, Bunn HF: Regulation of the erythropoietin gene: evidence that the oxygen sensor is a heme protein. Science 1988 (242):1412-1415

54   Law ML, Cai C-H, Lin F-K, Wei A, Huang S-Z, Hartz J-H, Morse H, Lin C-H, Jones C, Kao F-T: Chromosomal assignment of the human erythropoietin gene and its DNA polymorphism. Proc Natl Acad Sci USA 1986 (83):6920-6924

55   Ganser A, Bergmann M, Voelkers B, Gruetzmacher P, Scigalla P, Hoelzer D: In vivo effects of recombinant human erythropoietin on circulating human haematopoietic progenitor cells. Exp Hematol 1989 (17):433-435

56   Geissler K, Stockenhuber F, Kabrna E, Hinterberger W, Balcke P, Lecher K: Recombinant human erythropoietin and haematopoietic progenitor cells in vivo. Blood 1989 (73):2229

57   Oster W: Personal communicaton

58   Adamson JW: The promise of recombinant human erythropoietin. Sem Hematol 1989 (26):5-8

59   Eschbach JW, Egrie JC, Downing MR, Browne JK, Adamson JW: Correction of the anaemia of end-stage renal disease with recombinant human erythropietin. N Engl J Med 1987 (316):73-80

60   Lim VS, DeGowin RL, Zavala D, Kirchner PT, Abels R, Perry P, Fangman J: Recombinant human erythropoietin treatment in pre-dialysis patients. Ann Int Med 1989 (110):108-114

61   Oster W, Herrmann F, Cicco A, Gamm H, Zeile G, Brune T, Lindemann A, Schulz G, Mertelsmann R: Erythropoietin prevents chemotherapy-induced anemia. Blut 1989 (59):1-5

62   Oster W, Herrmann F, Gamm H, Zeile G, Lindemann A, Müller G, Brune T, Kraemer H-P, Mertelsmann R: Erythropoietin (EPO) for the treatment of anemia of malignancy due to neoplastic bone marrow infiltration. J Clin Oncol (in press)

63   Yang Y-C, Ciarletta AB, Temple PA, Chung MP, Kovacic S, Witek-Giannotti JS, Leary AC, Kirz R, Donahue RE, Wong GG, Clark SC: Human IL-3 (multi-CSF): identification by expression cloning of a novel hematopoietic growth factor related to murine IL-3. Cell 1986 (47):3-10

64   Donahue RE, Wang EA, Stone DK, Kamen R, Wong GG, Sehgal PK, Nathan DG, Clark SC: Stimulation of hematopoiesis in primates by continuous infusion of recombinant human GM-CSF. Nature 1986 (321):872-875

65   Welte K, Bonilla MA, Gillio AP, Boone TC, Potter GK, Gabrilove JL, Moore MAS, O'Reilley, Souza LM: Recombinant human G-CSF: Effects on hematopoiesis in normal and cyclophosphamide treated primates. J Exp Med 1987 (165):941-948

66   Ganser A, Lindemann A, Seipelt G, Ottmann OG, Herrmann F, Schulz G, Mertelsmann R, Hoelzer D: Effect of recombinant human Interleukin-3 (rhIL-3) in patients with bone marrow failure - a phase I/II trial. Blood 1989 (74): Abstr 177

67   Stanley ER, Hansen G, Woodcock J, Metcalf D: Colony stimulating factor and the regulation of granulopoiesis and macrophage production. Fed Proc 1975 (34):2272-2278

68   Howard M, Matis L, Malek TR, Shevach E, Kehl W, Cohen D, Nakanishi K, Paul WE: Interleukin-2 induces antigen reative T cell lines to secrete BCGF-1. J Exp Med 1983 (158):2024-2039

69   Nedwin GE, Svedersky LP, Bringman TS, Palladino MA, Goeddel DV: Effect of Interleukin-2, y-interferon, and mitogens on the production of tumor necrosis factor alpha and beta. J Immunol 1985 (135):2492-2497

70   Farrar WL, John HM, Farrar J: Regulation of the production of immune interferon and cytotoxic T-lymphocytes by IL-2. J Immumol 1981 (126):1120-1125

71   Kawase I, Brooks CG, Kuribayashi K, Olabunenaga S, Newman W, Gillis S, Henney CS: Interleukin-2 induces y-interferon production: Participation of macrophages and NK-like cells. J Immunol 1983 (131):288-292

72   Black CM, Catterall JR, Remington, JS: In vivo and in vitro activation of alveolar macrophages by recombinant y-Interferon. J Immunol 1987 (138):491-495

73   Murray HW, Spitalney GL, Nathan CF: Activation of mouse peritoneal macrophages in vitro and in vivo by y-Interferon. J Immunol 1985 (134):1619-1622

74   Nathan CF, Murray HW, Wiebe ME, Rubin BY: Identification of y-interferon as the lymphokine that activates human macrophage oxidative metabolism and antimicrobial activity. J Exp Med 1983 (158):670-689

75   Schreiber RD, Celada A: Molecular characterisation of y-interferon as a macrophage activating factor. In: Pick E (ed) Lymphokines. Academic Press, New York 1985 (11) pp 87-118

76   Malkovsky M, Loveland B, North M, Asherson GL, Gao L, Ward P, Fiers W: Recombinant interleukin-2 directly augments the toxicity of human monocytes. Nature 1987 (325):262-265

77   Phillips JH, Lanier LL: Dissection of the lymphokine-activated killer phenomenon. Relative contribution of peripheral blood natural killer cells and T lymphocytes to cytolysis. J Exp Med 1986 (164):814-825

78   Rosenberg SA, Mule JJ, Spiess PJ, Reichert CM, Schwarz SL: Regression of established pulmonary metastases and subcutaneous tumor mediated by the systemic administration of high-dose recombinant interleukin-2. J Exp Med 1985 (161):1169-1188

79 Rosenberg SA, Lotze MT, Muul LM, Leitman S, Chang AE, Ettinghausen SE, Matory YL, Skibber JM, Shilari E, Vetto JT, Seipp CA, Simpson C, Reichert CM: Observations on the systemic administration of autologous lymphokine-activated killer cells and recombinant interleukin-2 to patients with metastatic cancer. N Engl J Med 1985 (313):1485-1492

80 Rosenberg SA, Lotze MT, Muul LM, Chang AE, Avis FP, Leitman S, Linehan WM, Robertson CN, Lee RE, Rubin JT, Seipp CA, Simpson CG, White DE: A progress report on the treatment of 157 patients with advanced cancer using lymphokine-activated killer cells and interleukin-2 or high-dose interleukin-2 alone. N Engl J Med 1987 (316):889-879

81 West WH, Tauer KW, Yanelli JR, Marshall GD, Orr DW, Thurman GB, Oldham RK: Constant-infusion recombinant interleukin-2 in adoptive immunotherapy of cancer. N Engl J Med 1987 (316):898-905

82 Dutcher JP, Creekmore S, Weiss GR, Margolin K, Markowitz AB, Roper MA, Parkinson D: A phase II study of interleukin-2 and lymphokine activated killer cells in patients with metastatic malignant melanoma. J Clin Oncol 1989 (7):477-485

83 Fischer RI, Coltman CA, Doroshow JH, Rayner AA, Hawkins MJ, Mier JW, Wiernik P, McMannis JD, Weiss GR, Margolin KA, Gemlo BT, Hoth DF, Parkinson DR, Paietta E: Metastatic renal cell cancer treated with interleukin-2 and lymphokine-activated killer cells. A phase II clinical trial. Ann Int Med 1988 (108):518-523

84 Lotze MT, Matory YL, Rayner AA, Ettinghausen SE, Vetto JT, Seipp CA, Rosenberg SA: Clinical effects and toxicity of interleukin-2 in patients with cancer. Cancer 1986 (58):2764-2772

85 Gemlo BT, Palladino MA, Jaffe HS, Espevik TP, Rayner AA: Circulating cytokines in patients with metastatic cancer treated with recombinant interleukin 2 and lymphokine-activated killer cells. Cancer Res 1988 (48):5864-5867

86 Fraser-Scott K, Hatzakis H, Seong D, Jones CM, Wu KK: Influence of natural and recombinant interleukin 2 on endothelial cell arachidonate metabolism. Induction of de novo synthesis of prostaglandin H synthase. J Clin Invest 1988 (82):1877-1883

87 Mier JW, Vachino G, Van der Meer J, Numerof RP, Adams S, Cannon JG, Bernheim HA, Atkins MB, Parkinson DR, Dinarello CA: Induction of circulating tumor necrosis factor as the mechanism for the febrile response to interleukin-2 in cancer patients. J Clin Immunol 1988 (8):426-436

88 Lindemann A, Hoeffken K, Schmidt RE, Diehl V, Kloke O, Gamm H, Hayungs J, Oster W, Böhm M, Kolitz JE, Franks CR, Herrmann F, Mertelsmann R: A phase II study of low-dose cyclophosphamide and recombinant human interleukin-2 in metastatic renal cell carcinoma and malignant melanoma. Cancer Immunol Immunother 1989 (28):275-281

89 Mitchell MS: Low-dose cyclophosphamide and IL-2 in the treatment of advanced melanoma. In: Berger HG et al (eds) Cancer Therapy. Springer-Verlag, Berlin, Heidelberg 1989 pp 85-89

90 Mitchell MS, Kempf RA, Harel W, Shau H, Boswell WD, Lind S, Bradley EC: Effectiveness and tolerability of low-dose cyclophosphamide and low-dose intravenous interleukin-2 in disseminated melanoma. J Clin Oncol 1988 (6):409-424

91 Rosenberg SA, Packard BS, Aebersold PM, Solomon D, Topalian SL, Toy ST, Simon P, Lotze MT, Yang JC, Seipp CA, Simpson C, Carter C, Bock S, Schwartzenhuber D, Wei JP, White DE: Use of tumor-infiltrating lymphocytes and interleukin-2 in the immunotherapy of patients with metastatic melanoma. N Engl J Med 1988 (319):1676-1680

92 Bate CAW, Taverne J, Playfair JHL: Malarial parasites induce TNF production by macrophages. Immunol 1988 (64):227-231

93 Sayers TJ, Macker I, Chung J, Kugler E: The production of tumor necrosis factor by mouse bone marrow-derived macrophages in response to bacterial LPS and chemically synthesised monosaccharide precursors. J Immunol 1987 (138):2935-2940

94 Cuturi MC, Murphy M, Costa-Giomi MP, Weinmann R, Perussia B, Trinchieri G: Independent regulation of tumor necrosis factor and lymphotoxin production by human peripheral blood lymphocytes. J Exp Med 1987 (165):1581-1594

95 Degliantoni G, Murphy M, Kobayashi M, Francins MK, Perussia B, Trindieri G: Natural killer (NK) cell-derived hematopoietic colony inhibiting activity and NK cytotoxic factor: Relationship with tumor necrosis factor and synergisms with immune interferon. J Exp Med 1985 (162):1512-1530

96 Nedwin GE, Naylor SL, Sakaguchi AY, Smith D, Nedwin JJ, Pennica D, Goeddel DV, Gray PW: Human lymphotoxin and tumor necrosis factor genes. Stucture, homology and chromosomal location. Nucl Acids Res 1985 (13):6361-6373

97 Pennica D, Nedwin GE, Hayflick JS, Seeburg PH, Derynek R, Palladino MA, Kohr WJ, Aggarwl BB, Goeddel DV: Human tumor necrosis factor. Precursor, structure, expression and homology to lymphotoxin. Nature 1984 (312):724-729

98 Shalaby MR, Aggarwal BB, Rinderknecht E, Svedersky LP, Finkle BS, Palladino MA: Activation of human polymorphonuclear neutrophil functions by interferon-gamma and tumor necrosis factor. J Immunol 1985 (135): 2069-2073

99 Hori K, Ehrke MH, Mace K, Mihich E: Effect of recombinant tumor necrosis factor on tumoricidal activation of murine macrophages: synergism between tumor necrosis factor and y-interferon. Cancer Res 1987 (47):5868-5874

100 Ostensen ME, Thiele DL, Lipsky PE: Tumor necrosis factor alpha enhances cytolytic activity of human natural killer cells. J Immunol 1987 (138):4185-4191

101 Old LJ: Tumor necrosis factor (TNF). Science 1985 (230):630-632

102 Collins T, Lapierre LA, Fiers W, Strominger JL, Prober JS: Recombinant human tumor necrosis factor increases mRNA levels and surface expression of HLA-A,B antigens in vascular endothelial cells and dermal fibroblasts in vitro. Proc Nat Acad Sci (Wash) 1986 (83):446-450

103 Pohlman TH, Stanness KA, Beatty PG, Ochs HD, Harlan JM: An endothelial cell surface factor(s) induced in vitro by lipopolysaccharide, interleukin-1 and tumor necrosis factor-alpha increases neutophil adherence by a CDw 18-independent mechanism. J Immunol 1986 (135):4548-4533

104 Van De Wiel PA, Pieters RHH, Bloksma N: Synergistic action of recombinant TNF and endotoxin on cultured endothelial cells. Immunobiol 1987 (175):75

105 Leibovich SJ, Polverini PJ, Shephard MJ, Wiseman MJ, Shively DM, Nuseir V: Macrophage-induced angiogenesis is mediated by tumor necrosis factor alpha. Nature 1987 (329):630-632

106 Sugarman BJ, Aggarwal BB, Hass PE, Figari IS, Palladino MA, Shepard HM: Recombinant human tumor necrosis factor-alpha: effects on proliferation of normal and transformed cells. Science 1985 (230):943-945

107 Carswell EA, Old LJ, Kassel RL, Green S, Fiore D, Williamson B: An endotoxin induced serum factor that causes necrosis of tumors. Proc Natl Acad Sci (USA) 1975 (72):3666-3670

108 Haranaki K, Carswell EA, Williamson B, Pentergast JS, Satomi N, Old LJ: Purification, characterisation and antitumor activity of nonrecombinant mouse tumor necrosis factor . Proc Natl Acad Sci USA 1986 (83):3949-3953

109 Blick M, Sherwin SA, Rosenblum M, Gutterman J: Phase I study of recombinant tumor necrosis factor in cancer patients. Cancer Res 1987 (47):2986-2989

110 Mertelsmann R, Gamm H, Flener R, Herrmann F: Recombinant human tumor necrosis factor alpha (rhTNF-alpha) in advanced cancer: A phase I clinical trial. Proceedings of AACR 1987 (28): Abstr.1583

111 Bevilacqua MP, Pober JS, Mendrick DL, Cotram RS, Gimbrone MA: Identification of an inducible endothelial leukocyte adhesion molecule, E-LAM 1. Proc Nat Acad Sci (Wash) 1988 (in press)

112 Pober JS, Gimbrone MA, Lapierre LA, Mendrick DL, Fiers W, Rothlein R, Springer TA: Overlapping patterns of activation of human endothelial cells by interleukin-1, tumor necrosis factor and imune interferon. J Immunol 1986 (137):1893-1896

113 Haranaka K, Satomi N, Sakurai A, Haranaka R: Necrotizing activity of tumor necrosis factor and its mechanism. Ann Inst Pasteur/Immunol 1988 (139):288-294

114 Strander H: Anti-tumor effects of interferon and its possible use as an anti-neoplastic agent in man. Texas Rep Biol Med 1977 (35):429

115 Herberman RB, Ortaldo JR, Mantovani A, Hobbs DS, Kung HF, Pestka S: Effect of human recombinant interferon on cytotoxic activity of natural killer (NK) cells and monocytes. Cell Immunol 1982 (67):160-167

116 Lindahl P, Gresser I, Leary P et al: Enhanced expression of histocompatibility antigens of lymphoid cells treated with interferon. J Infect Dis 1976 (133 Suppl):A66

117 Brodeur BR, Merigan TC: Mechamism of the suppressive effect of interferon on antibody synthesis in vivo. J Immunol 1975 (114):1323-1328

118 Schnaper HW, Aune TM, Pierce CW: Suppressor T cell activation by human leukocyte interferon. J Immunol 1983 (131):2301-2306

119 Vilcek J, Gray PW, Rinderknecht E, Sevastopoulos CG: Interferon-y: A lymphokine for all seasons. In: Pick E (ed) Lymphokines. Academic Press, New York 1985 (11) pp 1-32

120 Quesada JR, Keuben J, Manning JJ, Hersh EM, Gutterman JU: Alpha interferon for induction of remission in hairy cell leukemia. N Engl J Med 1984 (310):15-18

121 Talpaz M, Kantarjian HM, McCredie K, Trujillo JM, Keating MJ, Gutterman JU: Hematologic remission and cytogenetic improvement induced by recombinant human interferon alpha in chronic myelogenous leukemia. N Engl J Med 1986 (314):1065-1069

122 Groopman JE, Gottlieb MS, Godman J, Hisugasu RT, Conant MA, Prince H, Faney JU, Derezin M, Weinstein WM, Casavante C, Rothman J, Rudnik SA, Volberding PA: Recombinant alpha-2-interferon therapy for Kaposi's sarcoma associated with acquired immunodeficiency syndrome. Ann Intern Med 1984 (100):671-676

123 Creagan ET, Ahmann DL, Green SJ, Long HJ, Frytak S, O'Fallon JR, Itri LM: Phase II study of recombinant leukocyte A interferon in disseminated malignant melanoma. J Clin Oncol 1984b (2):1002-1005

124 Niederle N, Kummer G: The role of interferon in the management of patients with hairy cell leukemia and multiple myeloma. In: Berger HG et al (eds):Cancer Therapy. Springer-Verlag, Berlin, Heidelberg 1989 pp 112-123

125 Aulitzky W, Gastl G, Tilg H, v. LHttichau I, Flener R, Huber C: Recurrence of hairy cell leukemia upon discontinuation of IFN treatment. Blut 1986 (53):215

126 Porzsolt F, Digel W, Buck C, Raghavachar A, Stefanic M, Schöniger W: Possible mechanism of interferon action in hairy cell leukemia. In: Berger HG et al (eds) Cancer Therapy. Springer-Verlag, Berlin, Heidelberg 1989 pp 126-131

127 Lindemann A, Ludwig WD, Oster W, Mertelsmann R, Herrmann F: High level secretion of TNF-alpha contributes to hematopoietic failure in hairy cell leukemia. Blood 1989 (73):880-884

128 Talpaz M, Kantarjian H, Kurzrock R, Trujillo JM, Gutterman JU: Sustained complete cytogenetic response among Philadelphia positive chronic myelogenous leukemia (CML PH1) patients treated with alpha interferon. Blood 1989 (74): Abstr 289

129 Higano CS, Raskind W, Durnam D, Singer JW: Alpha interferon (IF) induces cytogenetic remissions in patients who relapse with chronic myelogenous leukemia (CML) after allogenic bone marrow transplantation (BMT). Blood 1989 (74): Abstr 307

130 Kantarjian H, Keating M, McCredie K, Gutterman J, Freireich E, Deisseroth A, Talpaz M: Treatment of advanced stages of Philadelphia-chromosome (Ph)-positive chronic myelogenous leukemia (CL) with alpha interferon (IFN-alpha) and low-dose cytosine arabinoside (Ara-C). Blood 1989 (4): Abstr 878

131 Jones GJ, Itri LM: Safety and tolerance of recombbinant interferon alpha-2a (Roferon-A) in cancer patients. Cancer 1986 (57):1709-1715

132 Bunn PA, Foon KA, Ihde DC, Longo DL, Eddy J, Winkler CF, Weach SR, Zeffren J, Sherwins S, Oldham R: Recombinant leukocyte A interferon: an active agent in advanced cutaneous T-cell lymphomas. Ann Int Med 1984 (101):484-487

133 Foon KA, Sherwin SA, Abrams PG, Kongo DU, Fer MF, Stevenson HC, Ochs JJ, Bottino GC, Schoenberger CS, Zeffren J, Jaffe ES, Oldhorn RK: Treatment of advanced Non-Hodgkin's lymphoma with recombinant leukocyte A interferon. N Engl J Med 1984 (311):1148-1152

134 Einzig AI, Krown SE, Oettgen HF: Recombinant leukocyte A interferon (rIFNa-A) in renal cell cancer (RCC). Proc Am Soc Clin Oncol 1984 (3): Abstr C-209

Mechanisms of T-Cell Activation

Hermann Wagner and Klaus Heeg

Institute of Medical Microbiology and Hygiene, Technical University of Munich, Trogerstrasse 9, 8000 Munich, FRG

T lymphocytes develop and mature within the thymus gland [1]. It seems likely that the thymus has evolved as a site for the provision of efficient signalling of T-cell maturation. In addition, recent studies have indicated the importance of antigen expression (especially expression of self-MHC antigens) by the thymic environment in shaping the T-cell receptor repertoire by positive selection, i.e., selection of T cells with useful receptors, and negative selection, i.e., removal of potentially autoreactive cells [2].

Cell Surface Structures Involved in T-Cell Activation

Morphologically similar to B cells, T cells also express surface receptors for antigens. As in B cells, gene DNA segments undergo rearrangement in T cells. Unlike antigen receptors of B cells that represent membrane-bound immunoglobulins, antigen receptors of T cells are neither secreted, nor do they bind soluble antigen [3]. Classical T cells express α/β heterodimers as antigen receptors [3]. In the peripheral, recirculating T-cell pool, there exists an additional minor set (2-5 %) of T lymphocytes expressing γ/δ heterodimers as antigen receptor [4]. The specificity and function of the latter T-cell subset is, as yet, largely unknown.

The antigen receptor on T lymphocytes recognises foreign antigens in association with products of the major histocompatibility complex (MHC) locus, a phenomenon called MHC-restriction [5]. In fact, MHC molecules are now considered as a special transport system in antigen-presenting cells (APC), which function as receptors for antigenic peptides generated from denatured or processed proteins. Consequently, antigenic peptides are rescued from extensive intracellular digestion and are subsequently exposed as a MHC-peptide complex to T cells. Two apparently independent MHC transport systems exist, one pathway operating via class I MHC molecules, and another via class II MHC molecules. Both pathways appear to be independent of each other. The class II MHC presentation pathway transports foreign peptides derived from exogenous sources - either proteins that are internalised and processed in endosomes, or peptides that are in circulation and bind directly to surface MHC molecules. In contrast, the class I MHC molecules bind peptides from endogenous sources, i.e., peptides derived from proteins that are synthesised and assembled in the endoplasmatic reticulum (ER).

As stated above, in order to generate the sequence diversity necessary to recognise the many antigens (peptides), the T-cell receptor (TCR) genes undergo somatic DNA rearrangements. Since these rearrangements appear to be random, one can surmise that certain combinations of the TCRs may be self-recognising, and thus potentially autoreactive. Results obtained in TCR-transgenic mouse model systems have been informative in this respect [2]. Using clonotypic antibodies to track the fate of developing T cells expressing a given TCR, compelling evidence has been provided that self-tolerance to self-MHC antigens present in the thymus is accomplished by clonal deletion (usually termed negative selection) [6]. On the other hand, developing thymocytes appear to interact with self-MHC molecules as part of normal differentiation. In fact, this interaction appears to be MHC-allele specific and mandatory [7]. If one assumes that, at a distinct stage of development, thymocytes are uniquely susceptible to signals received via weak TCR interaction with MHC gene products expressed on thymic epithelial cells, thymocytes with the appropriate TCR may, in fact, be induced to proliferate (instead of being paralysed), a process resulting in positive selection.

The process of antigen recognition by T cells involves the physical interaction of a TCR with a nominal peptide antigen bound to a specific MHC molecule (often referred to as restricting element). This process, i.e., T-cell activation as a consequence of TCR binding to the peptide-MHC complex, is, in general, not only dictated by the TCR complex itself, but, rather, dependent on other structures, often referred to as adhesion molecules [8]. These adhesion molecules include CD4, CD8 and lymphocyte-function-associated antigen 1 (LFA-1). CD4 and CD8 structures bind to monomorphic regions of class II and class I MHC structures, respectively, thereby facilitating the specific interaction of the TCR with the peptide-presenting MHC molecule [9]. In addition, the CD2/LFA-3 receptor-ligand pair facilitates non-antigen-specific interactions between T lymphocytes and their cognate partners [10]. To date, T cell activation can be viewed as a 3-step event (Fig. 1). Accordingly, CD2/LFA-3 as well as LFA-3/ICAM-1 pairing provides a basis for cell-cell conjugate formation (physical interaction between the T cell and the antigen presenting cell (APC)). In the second step, CD4/monomeric class II MHC interactions (or CD8/monomeric class I MHC interactions) add further to stabilising cell-cell conjugate formation. The subsequent cross-linking of TCRs by an array of antigenic peptide-MHC complexes results in specific T-cell activation. Under physiologic conditions, the APC fulfills these requirements because it expresses multiple peptide-bound MHC molecules, in addition to LFA-3 and the counter receptor for

Distinct Steps in Antigen Recognition

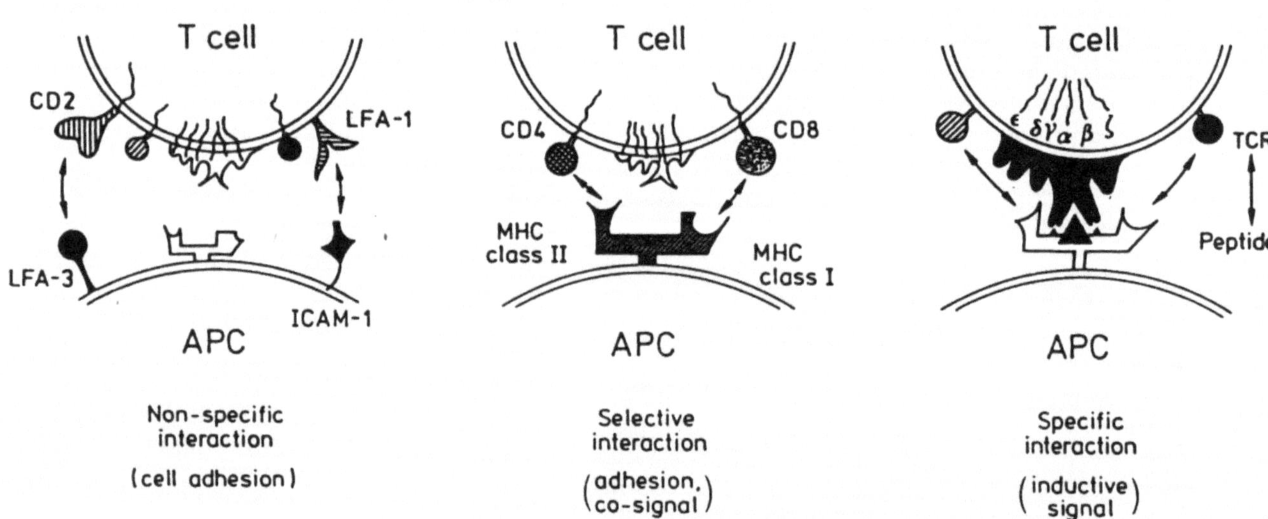

Fig. 1. T cell triggering is viewed as a 3-step event. In a first step, receptor-ligand pairs of adhesion molecules (CD2/LFA-3; LFA-1/ICAM-1) cause unspecific cell-cell adhesion between the antigen-reactive T cell and the APC. This cell adhesion is strengthened in a second step by receptor-ligand pairing of CD4 with class II MHC molecules (or CD8 with class I MHC molecules). Finally, the α/ß TCR binds to antigenic peptides (triangle) as presented by the MHC molecule (ß-sheet with 2 α-helices bordering the ß-sheet in a table-like fashion). Intracellular signalling initiated by cross-linking of the α/ß TCRs involves the T3 complex (T3 γ, δ, ε, ζ chain)

LFA-1, namely ICAM-1. It is likely that stabilisation of conjugate formation between antigen-reactive T cells and respective APCs promoted by adhesion molecules reduces the number of TCR-antigenic peptide/MHC comlexes required to attain a T-cell activation threshold. However, mere physical facilitation of cell-cell conjugate formation would not allow the latter conclusion. In fact, CD4, CD8 and CD2 structures contain cytoplasmatic parts, which, in turn, are associated with a lymphocyte-specific protein-tyrosine kinase termed p56^{lck} [11]. It may therefore be postulated that receptor-ligand interaction of CD4, CD8, or CD2 modulates p56^{lck} activity, thus complementing T-cell activation signals caused by TCR cross-linking [12].

T-T-Cell Interactions in T-Cell Mediated Responses

Within mature recirculating T cells expressing α/ß TCR structures, the expression of CD4 and CD8 cell surface structures is mutually exclusive. Since there is no evidence that the use of Vα and Vß TCR segments differs in CD4+CD8- and CD8+CD4- T cells, it follows that the CD4 (or CD8) molecules determine whether the T-cell subset recognises antigenic peptides in the context of class II (or class I) MHC molecules [13]. Upon activation, either the CD4+ or the CD8+ subset can produce lymphokines, although CD4+ T cells are primarily associated with T-helper function, i.e., lymphokine secretion, whilst CD8+ T cells primarily mount antigen-specific cytotoxic effector functions [14]. In mice, CD4+ helper T cells (Th) can even be subdivided according to their pattern of lymphokine secretion [15]. Thus, Th-1 CD4+ T cells produce IL2 and IFN-γ and thus mediate delayed-type hypersensitivity, while Th-2 CD4+T cells produce IL4 and IL5, and thus stimulate antibody production. In the human system, however, the lymphokine production profile of a given CD4+ T cell line appears not to be stable but dependent on the activation stimuli used.

Lymphokine Requirements for the Primary Activation of Murine CD8+ T Cells

Primary activation of the resting CD8+ T cells consists of two distinctly regulated phases, termed competence and progression. Competence signals are delivered by antigen (peptide) presented via professional APCs such as dentritic cells (see Fig. 1), thereby inducing receptors for a variety of lymphokines. Binding of autocrine- or paracrine-secreted growth- and differentiation-promoting lymphokines then causes progression, i.e., growth and differentiation into effector T cells. While there is ample evidence that each lymphokine performs multiple functions (pleiotropy), dependent on the respective target cell, it is also becoming clear that there is a certain redundancy, i.e., more than one lymphokine can mediate identical functions.

As mentioned above, TCRs recognise conjugates of antigenic peptides and MHC molecules; however, this binding is not sufficient to induce competence in resting T cells. Therefore, additional inductive signals are necessary and may be provided by accessory molecules such as CD4, CD8 or CD2. To bypass the need for APCs, we resorted, in the past, to the use of solid-phase anti-TCR monoclonal antibodies (Mab) to efficiently initiate competence induction in murine CD8+ T cells via strong cross-linking of their TCRs. In addition, we plated highly purified resting CD8+ T cells at low cell densities (< 1000 cells/culture) in order to minimise the likelihood of contaminating cells.

Interestingly, when resting CD8+ T cells are triggered by solid-phase anti-TCR Mab, the expression of IL2 receptors (IL2R) is greatly upregulated by rec. IL2 added. Yet the IL2R+ CD8+ T cells are weakly driven into the cell cycle by IL2. Responsiveness is brought about by a macrophage-derived cytokine, which turned out to be IL6. Neither IL1, IL3, IL4, IFN-γ nor TNF-α were effective. In this system, IL6 acted as a competence factor by conveying IL2 resposiveness to IL2R+ preactivated CD8+ T cells [16].

In line with others [17], we observed that IL4 acts as an autonomous growth factor, the signal pathway being independent of that used by IL2 [18]. However, at the cellular level both the IL2- and the IL4-driven progression pathways appear to be interconnected [19]. Firstly, in combination, IL4 and IL2 greatly augment the proliferative and differentiative (cytolytic) response generated. Secondly, at low concentrations IL4 synergises with IL2. Thirdly, IL4 inhibits the decay of IL2 reponsiveness by delaying the loss of high-affinity IL2R. Interestingly, IL4 not only induces cell growth but selectively augments, in a dose-dependent fashion, the lytic activity of differentiating CTLs. The differentiative (cytotoxicity inducing) action of IL4 acts late, and within 24 hours prior to the ^{51}Cr-cytotoxicity assay.

The immunosuppressive drug cyclosporine (CsA) affects primary T-cell activation by blocking TCR-mediated signalling of lymphokine gene transcription, such as that for IL2, as well as that for IL4. In addition, CsA does not block the expression of IL2R but the acquisition of sensitivity to IL2 and IL4 during primary activation of CD8+ T cells [20]. As described above, the IL4- and IL2-driven signal pathways synergise with each other, and thus are interconnected. This might explain our unexpected finding that, in the presence of IL2 and IL4, the CsA-mediated immunesuppression is selective in the sense that highly cytotoxic CD8+ T cells are generated in primary mixed lymphocyte reactions towards class I MHC incompatible stimulator cells in the virtual absence of cell proliferation [20]. Obviously, cell growth (clonal expansion) appears to be CsA sensitive, while the IL4-driven differentiation of resting CD8+ T cells in cytolytic T effector cells appears to be CsA resistant.

Lymphokine Secretion and Expression of Cytolytic Activity by Clonally Defined CD8+ T Cells

Although activated CD4+ T cells are the principal source of lymphokines, it is clear that also activated murine CD8+ T cells produce lymphokines such as IL2 [21,22]. In analysing clonally developing CD8+ T cells responding either to ConA, allogenic class I MHC antigens, or TNP-conjugated syngeneic MHC antigens, we have observed a clear-cut segregation of those colonies producing IL2 from those exhibiting cytolytic activity [22]. In fact, both functions appeared to exclude each other, and bifunctional clones were the exception to the rule. When, however, the activation protocol was experimentally divided into a step "competence induction" and a step "induction of progression", i.e., resting CD8+ T cells were first induced with the mitogen ConA and subsequently, after washing off ConA, clonal growth was sustained by IL2 in the absence of ConA, then the great majority of clonally developing colonies were bifunctional, i.e., they secreted IL2 and exhibited cytolytic functions as well. Note that, upon addition of ConA in the second-step culture which contained additional IL2, clonal segregation of both functions reappeared. Obviously, clonally developing CD8+ T cells do have the potential to be bifunctional. We conclude that it is the nature of the T cell stimuli used for activation which determines the set of final functions expressed.

Conclusion

To complement TCR-antigen interactions, the competence phase of resting T-cells is controlled by additional, non-specific, receptor-ligand interaction facilitating cell-cell adhesion. While IL6 acts as competence factor by conveying IL2 responsiveness to IL2R+ CD8+ T cells, both IL2 and IL4 function as growth factors. It is the nature of T cell stimuli used which determines the set of functions released in clonally developing CD8+ T cells.

Acknowledgement

We thank Drs. T. Miethke and J. Schmitt for sharing their results with us.

REFERENCES

1   Miller JFP and Osoba D: Current concepts of immunological function of thymus. Physiol Rev 1967 (47):437-487

2   von Boehmer H, Teh HS and Kisielow P: The thymus selects the useful, neglects the useless, and destroys the harmful. Immunol Today 1989 (10):57-61

3   Hedrik SM, Cohen DI, Nielson EA and Davies MM: Isolation of cDNA clones encoding T cell specific membrane-associated proteins. Nature 1984 (308):145-148

4   Hayday AC, Saito H, Gilles SD, Kranz DM, Tonigawa G, Eisen HN and Tonegawa S: Structure, organization and somatic rearrangement of T cell gamma genes. Cell 1985 (40):259-269

5   Bjorkman PJ, Saper MA, Samraour B, Bennet WS, Strominger JL and Wiley DC: The foreign antigen binding site and T cell recognition regions of class I histocompatibility antigens. Nature 1987 (329):506-512

6   Kappler J, Roehm N and Marrack P: T cell tolerance by clonal elimination in the thymus. Cell 1987 (49):273-280

7   Marrack P, Lo D, Brinster R, Palmiter R, Bunkly L, Flavell RH and Kappler JW: The effect of thymus environment on T cell development and tolerance. Cell 1988 (53):627-634

8   Springer TA, Dustin ML, Kishimoto TK, and Marlin SD: The lymphocyte function-associated LFA-1, CD2 and LFA-3 molecules: cell adhesion receptors of the immune system. Ann Rev Immunol 1987 (5):223-252

9   Parnes JR: Molecular biology and function of CD4 and CD8. Adv Immunol 1989 (44):265-311

10 Shaw S, Luce G, Quinones R, Gress RE, Springer TA and Sanders ME: Two antigen-independent adhesion pathways used by human cytotoxic T cell clones. Nature 1986 (323):262-264

11 Alexander DR and Cantrell DA: Kinases and phosphatases in T cell activation. Immunol Today 1989 (10):200-205

12 Barber EK, Dasgupta JD, Schlossmann SF, Trevillyau JM and Rudd CE: The CD4 and CD8 antigens are coupled to a protein-tyrosine kinase (p56^{lck}) that phosphorylates the CD3 complex. Proc Natl Acad Sci USA 1989 (86):3277-3281

13 Bach F, Widmer M, Segall M, Bach M and Klein J: Genetic and immunological complexity of major histocompatibility regions. Science 1978 (176):1024-1037

14 Wagner H and Röllinghoff M: T-T cell interactions during in vitro cytotoxic allograft responses. I. Soluble products from Lyt1$^+$ cells trigger autonomously antigen-primed Lyt2, 3$^+$ T cells to proliferation and cytolytic activity. J Exp Med 1978 (148):1523-1529

15 Mosmann TC and Coffman RL: Heterogeneity of cytokine secretion patterns and function of helper T cells. Adv Immunol 1989 (46):111-147

16 Schmidberger R, Miethke T, Heeg K and Wagner H: Primary activation of murine CD8 T cells via crosslinking of T3 cell surface structures: Two signals regulate induction of interleukin 2 responsiveness. Eur J Immunol 1988 (18):277-282

17 Widmer MB and Grabstein KH: Regulation of cytolytic T lymphocyte generation by B cell stimulatory factor. Nature 1987 (326):795-798

18 Miethke T, Schmidberger R, Heeg K, Gillis S and Wagner H: Interleukin 4 (BSF-1) induces growth in resting murine CD8$^+$ T cells triggered via crosslinking of T3 cell surface structures. Eur J Immunol 1988 (18):767-772

19 Bubeck R, Miethke T, Heeg K and Wagner H: Synergy between interleukin 4 and interleukin 2 conveys resistance to cyclosporine A during primary in vitro activation of murine CD8 cytotoxic T cell precursors. Eur J Immunol 1989 (19):625-630

20 Heeg K, Gillis S and Wagner H: Interleukin 4 bypasses the immune suppressive effect of cyclosporine A (CsA) during the in vitro induction of murine cytotoxic T lymphocytes. J Immunol 1988 (141):2330-2334

21 Singer A, Muritz TE, Golding H, Rosenberg A and Mizuocki T: Recognition requirements for the activation, differentiation and function of T-helper cells specific for class I MHC alloantigens. Immunol Rev 1987 (98):143-170

22 Heeg K, Steeg C, Schmitt J and Wagner H: Identification of interleukin 2 producing T helper cells within murine Lyt2$^+$ T lymphocytes: frequency, specificity and clonal segregation from Lyt2$^+$ precursors of cytotoxic T lymphocytes. J Immunol 1987 (138):4121-4127

Characteristics of LAK Cells and Their Use in Adoptive Therapy of Cancer in Experimental Animals

Ronald B. Herberman

Pittsburgh Cancer Institute and Departments of Medicine and Pathology, University of Pittsburgh, School of Medicine, Pittsburgh, PA 15213, U.S.A.

Proliferation and Activation of NK Cells by IL2

Interleukin 2 (IL2) has been the main factor that has been focused on for *in vitro* expansion and strong activation of NK cells. As with T cells, this proliferative effect of IL2 on NK cells has been shown to be dependent on an interaction of the lymphokine with receptors for IL2, as detected by anti-Tac monoclonal antibodies [1]. Proliferating LGL have been shown to express Tac and anti-Tac completely interfered with the growth of the cells and their maintenance of cytotoxic activity. However, as a major divergence from the data obtained with T cells, in which IL2 receptors had to be induced by mitogens or antigens in order for the cells to become responsive to IL2 [2], IL2 alone has been shown to promote the growth of human or murine NK cells [1,3]. Quite unexpectedly, fresh IL2-responsive human LGL were found to have no detectable IL2 receptors, as measured either by flow cytometry with anti-Tac or by binding studies with radiolabelled anti-Tac [1]. In addition, messenger RNA for IL2 receptors was not detectable in fresh human LGL [1]. However, upon exposure of such LGL to IL2 alone, message for the Tac receptor became detectable within 2 days of culture and this was accompanied by detectable expression of Tac receptors on the cells and the onset of proliferation. Thus, it appears that IL2 alone can induce the upregulation of Tac receptors at the transcriptional level [1] and this appears to account for the ability of this lymphokine by itself to promote the growth of NK cells.

The ability of IL2 to directly stimulate NK cells [4] appears to be due to constitutive expression of the p70 beta chain of the IL2 receptor. The combination of the alpha chain (Tac) with the beta chain has been shown to lead to high-affinity IL2 receptors. In recent studies with rat NK cells, proliferation as well as activation have been found to occur with continued expression only of the beta chain of the IL2 receptor (Hiserodt, Capar and DeLeo, personal communication). Monoclonal antibodies against purified IL2-activated rat NK cells blocked proliferation of the cells and appear to detect the non-Tac-related beta chain receptor for IL2 on rat NK cells.

Lymphokine-activated killer (LAK) cells have been described [5] that share many of the characteristics of NK cells. LAK cells have been activated after a short period of culture *in vitro* with highly purified IL2 and display cytotoxic activity against a variety of autologous, allogeneic and xenogeneic tumours. These cells were initially thought to lack markers typical of fresh NK cells, to be devoid of cytolytic activity prior to culture, and to develop T cell markers upon activation [6]. However, more recent studies in several laboratories have indicated that most LAK activity developing from blood or splenic lymphocytes is attributable to IL2-stimulated NK cells and, in fact, most LAK cells and their progenitors have a phenotype characteristic of NK cells but not T cells [7].

In the initial descriptions of LAK cells, much emphasis was placed on the observations that fresh solid tumour target cells appeared to be insusceptible to lysis by NK cells [5]. However, susceptibility or resistance of target cells to lysis by NK cells appears to be a relative rather than an absolute distinction. Under some circumstances, "NK-resistant" targets can be lysed to a significant extent by unstimulated NK cells. Regarding the possibility of NK activity against fresh noncultured tumour cells, low but significant levels of cytotoxic activity against fresh human leukaemia cells were observed in the earliest studies of human NK cells [8]. Similarly, some of the "NK-resistant" culture cell lines that are being used as good targets for assessing LAK activity, particularly the Raji cell line, were used in early studies of NK activity [9,10], prior to the discovery of more sensitive targets such as K562. Clearly, the increase of NK activity by various agents, including interferon as well as IL2, can not only increase the levels of reactivity against NK-sensitive target cells but can also induce detectable levels of lysis of targets that seemed refractory to unstimulated NK cells. The artificiality of the distinction between NK-sensitive and NK-resistant target cells has been emphasised by a series of *in vivo* studies of the role of NK cells in resistance to metastatic spread of tumours. Much of the strong evidence for the potent ability of NK cells *in vivo* to rapidly eliminate tumour cells from the circulation and to prevent the subsequent development of metastases in the lungs and other organs has come from studies with tumour cell lines which appear to be highly resistant to NK activity *in vitro* [11,12,13].

Even when it has not been possible to detect lysis of fresh leukaemia or solid tumour target cells by unseparated blood or splenic lymphocytes, significant levels of NK activity could be detected simply after purification of the effector cells. Human LGL, purified by Percoll density gradient centrifugation, have been shown to have significant cytotoxic activity against the majority of fresh solid tumour cells or fresh leukaemia cells tested. The effector cells for solid tumour targets appeared to be a subset of LGL [14], but in conjugate assays with 2 target cells it was shown that the effector cells lysing autologous tumour cells also could lyse the NK-sensitive K562 cell line [15]. The effector cells reactive against human leukaemia targets were further shown to be CD16+ and CD56+ (NKH1+

or Leu 19+) [16,17]. In contrast to such lytic activity of LGL against fresh human "NK-resistant" targets, LGL-depleted populations of small T cells were without detectable activity.

In addition to the above evidence that unstimulated NK cells as well as LAK cells can have cytotoxic activity against fresh tumour cells and other "NK-resistant" targets, there are some indications that NK cells and LAK cells may recognise the same target structures. In cold target inhibition experiments, NK-susceptible targets such as K562 could efficiently inhibit human LAK activity against an NK-resistant target. Similarly, NK-sensitive target cells were found to adsorb LAK cells more efficiently in monolayer depletion experiments than did NK-resistant cells. Further, after exposure of NK-susceptible target cells to LAK cells, the surviving target cells were found to be transiently resistant to both NK cells and cells with LAK activity [18]. One might explain such data by postulating that NK-sensitive target cells simply express NK target structures better or in higher concentration than NK-resistant targets. However, to satisfactorily settle this question, it will be necessary to directly characterise the target structures recognised by NK cells and LAK cells and in, a complementary way, characterise the recognition structures on each type of effector cells.

Extensive studies have now been done on the phenotype of both the lymphocytes which develop LAK activity after culture with IL2 (i.e., progenitors of cells with LAK activity) and the effector cells themselves, after culture in the presence of IL2. Although the initial studies on LAK activity suggested a shift in phenotype, from progenitors lacking T cell as well as NK cell markers [6] to effector cells with T cell markers, subsequent studies have indicated the expression of a very similar pattern of markers on both the progenitors and effector cells. Data on the phenotype of LAK cells have now been obtained in 3 species (mouse and rat as well as human), and these are summarised below.

With regard to the characteristics which have been associated with the blood or splenic lymphocytes which developed LAK activity after culture in the presence of IL2, the most extensive studies have been performed with human lymphocytes. It seems clear that most of the LAK activity from blood lymphocytes is generated from cells with the same characteristics as NK cells. The progenitors of LAK activity in human peripheral blood have been shown to be mainly LGL with the CD3⁻ CD16⁺ CD56⁺ phenotype. Some of the progenitors appear to be low-density lymphocytes which lack the characteristic granules of LGL and thereby are resistant to the lysosomotropic agent, L-leucine methyl ester [19]. Somewhat divergent data have been the finding of low levels of LAK activity generated from CD3⁺ blood lymphocytes. CD3⁺ CD56⁺ lymphocytes have been detected in low concentrations in peripheral blood, have been associated with some MHC-unrestricted cytotoxicity, and have been shown to give rise to some clones with "NK-like" activity [20,21]. More strongly divergent results have come from a recent study [22], indicating that appreciable LAK activity could be generated from a wide variety of lymphocyte subpopulations, including CD4⁺ and CD8⁺ T cells and also B cells. The explanation for these divergent results is not clear, but may be attributable to some technical limitations of the panning technique utilised for cell separations.

The LAK activity generated from mouse or rat spleen cells or bone marrow cells has been associated with progenitors with characteristics virtually identical to those associated with NK cells. For example, rat NK cells have been closely associated with LGL and the asialo GM_1 and CD8 cell surface antigens [23]. In addition, cell surface molecules reactive with polyclonal and monoclonal antibodies to laminin have been reported to be selectively expressed on rat NK cells [24]. These same markers have also been detected on the progenitors of rat LAK cells [25]. Furthermore, high levels of LAK activity was generated from highly purified populations of blood or splenic LGL, while little or no activity was generated from purified populations of T cells. Most studies with mouse lymphocytes have also indicated that the splenic progenitors of LAK activity have a phenotype compatible with NK cells, with expression of asialo GM_1, some positivity for Thy 1, and absence of L3T4 or Lyt2 [26]. In contrast, Shortman et al. [27] have depicted the generation from Lyt2⁺ cells of some mouse strains by a limiting dilution technique of cells

with lytic activity against NK-resistant targets. However, these cultures have been performed in the presence of Con A and irradiated killer cells and those conditions may account for the divergent results.

With regard to characteristics of cells with LAK activity, generated from blood or splenic lymphocytes upon culture in the presence of IL2, the phenotype of most of the progenitor cells and of most of the effectors for LAK activity is very similar, each quite compatible with the phenotype of NK cells but divergent from that of typical T cells. As with the progenitors of LAK activity, some effector cells with LAK activity have been shown to have T cell markers. However, under the usual conditions of generating LAK activity from blood or splenic lymphocytes, such effector cells appear to be very infrequent. Also, such T cells with LAK activity appear to have been derived from T cell progenitors. It is of interest that the CD3⁺ human lymphocytes with LAK activity appear to be, at least in part, atypical T cells expressing CD56 [21,28] but lacking expression of either CD4 or CD8 [29].

Thus, LAK should be considered a phenomenon rather than a new or distinct effector cell, with most of the blood or splenic activity attributable to NK cells. The LAK phenomenon appears to be of particular interest because of the potent ability of IL2 to both stimulate cytotoxic activity and to promote the expansion of the effector cell population.

Therapy of Tumours in Experimental Animals with IL2-Activated Effector Cells

The initial studies with normal lymphocytes cultured in the presence of IL2 indicated that such cells could have significant anti-tumour effects [30]. Normal murine lymphocytes cultured for 3 days in the presence of a high concentration of human recombinant IL2 were then shown to have significant therapeutic activity against metastases from various syngeneic sarcomas when injected intravenously at 3 and 6 days after tumour challenge, along with repeated high doses of human recombinant IL2 (25,000 units intraperitoneally 3 times a day from day 3 through 8). This treatment with high doses (10^8 cells) of LAK cells significantly reduced the number of metastases detectable in the lungs and liver but did not result in complete elimination of metastases or cures of the mice. Rosenberg and his colleagues [31,32] then began a series of focused efforts to optimise the parameters for effective therapy of syngeneic murine sarcomas by this approach. They examined several of the parameters of the treatment protocol to gain some insight into the requirements for effective therapy. Two injections of LAK cells, 3×10^7 or 10^8, were found to be more effective than one dose of cells. The cells cultured for 3 days in the presence of IL2 were shown to have optimal therapeutic effects, and it is of interest that this length of culture also resulted in peak levels of cytotoxic reactivity. Therapeutic effects were seen in recipients pretreated with 400 rad of radiation, suggesting that the therapeutic effects were not due to a major host component. In contrast, irradiation of the LAK cells with 3,000 rad resulted in a loss of efficacy, suggesting that the transferred cells had to not only remain viable but also be able to proliferate. However, since the transfer of allogeneic LAK cells appeared to be as effective as syngeneic cells, long-term survival and proliferation in the recipients was probably not required. The administration of recombinant IL2 along with LAK cells appeared to be required, with the presumption that the lymphokine treatment was needed for in vivo stimulation of proliferation of the donor cells. The use of 6,000 units of recombinant IL2 per dose together with LAK cells was highly effective, but 30,000 units per dose appeared to give better results. In contrast, the use of up to 34,000 units of recombinant IL2 per dose, without administration of LAK cells, had no detectable effect on tumour metastases when the treatment was initiated on day 3 after tumour challenge. However, 20,000 units of IL2 per dose was effective by itself in significantly reducing established pulmonary metastases when treatment was initiated at day 10 after tumour challenge. At both days 3 and 10, a total of 100,000 units per dose of IL2 were appreciably more effective. To understand the possible basis for the therapeutic effects of high doses of IL2 by itself and also to assess the hypothesis regarding the need for

administration of IL2 to support in vivo proliferation of transferred LAK cells, studies have been performed on the ability of various doses of recombinant IL2 to stimulate proliferation of lymphocytes in vivo. As a parallel to the dose of IL2 shown to be required for significant therapeutic effects of LAK cells, 6,000 units of IL2 administered intraperitoneally 3 times per day was found to significantly increase the uptake of radiolabelled iododeoxyuridine, as a measure of proliferating lymphocytes, in a variety of organs, including the lungs, liver, kidneys, and mesenteric lymph nodes [33]. Substantially higher levels of proliferation in these organs were observed after administration of 100,000 units of IL2 per dose. Although the cellular composition of the proliferating lymphocytes was not studied in detail, it is of note that augmented levels of cytotoxic reactivity against NK-resistant target cells were observed after the in vivo stimulation with IL2. As a further study along these lines, uptake of radiolabeled iododeoxyuridine was examined in mice treated with 6,000 units of IL2 per dose, alone or in combination with transferred LAK cells [34]. The combination of both treatments gave higher levels of proliferation in the lungs and liver, but in other organs such as spleen, kidneys and lymph nodes, the maximal uptake of radiolabelled material was observed with IL2 alone. As another correlation with the therapy studies, expansion of lymphocytes was also seen in recipients pretreated with 500 rad of radiation.

In the above series of studies, although adoptive immunotherapy could induce an impressive reduction in established metastases of murine sarcomas, the therapeutic effects were usually transient, and few, if any, complete cures were achieved. To further explore this approach to therapy and to explore the treatment conditions that might be required for curative results, a model of transplantable murine adenocarcinoma of the kidney (Renca) was developed [35]. By inoculation of Renca cells under the kidney capsule, a course of tumour progression was initiated that closely mimicked the progression of human renal cell carcinoma, with spontaneous metastases to regional lymph nodes in the peritoneal cavity, liver and lungs. This model has become of particular interest because of the recent clinical studies [36] indicating that adoptive immunotherapy with LAK cells plus recombinant IL2 may be particularly effective for metastatic renal cell carcinoma (see chapter by T. Hercend in this volume). In the initial therapy experiments, treatment was initiated 7 days after tumour challenge, when only occult metastases were present. Administration of cytotoxic lymphocytes, after 24 hours of incubation with human recombinant IL2, plus recombinant IL2, resulted in a significant increase in survival but only a low percentage of cures. Similarly, treatment at this time with chemotherapy, either doxorubicin or cyclophosphamide, gave a low percentage of cures. In contrast, combination chemoimmunotherapy with doxorubicin and IL2-stimulated cytotoxic lymphocytes plus IL2 resulted in a cure of two thirds of the tumour-bearing mice. These results are quite interesting from several standpoints: Firstly, they demonstrate that treatment with a combination of modalities may be considerably more effective than immunotherapy alone, with cytoreduction or other effects of chemotherapy leading to synergistic interactions with adoptive immunotherapy. Secondly, the protocol for immunotherapy that was required for these impressive results was considerably less intensive than those utilised by Mule and his colleagues [32]. The lymphocytes utilised for transfer were cultured with only 200 units of IL2 for a shorter period, only 24 hours, since these conditions were sufficient to induce strong cytotoxicity *in vitro* against Renca cells. The immunotherapy itself consisted of 3 daily intravenous inoculations of 3.5×10^7 cultured lymphocytes plus 3 daily intravenous inoculations of 10,000 units of IL2. These doses were lower than those utilised in the above-described experiments, indicating that under some circumstances effective therapy can be achieved with relatively modest doses of IL2 and cytotoxic lymphocytes.

Similar results were achieved when a combination of doxorubicin and IL2-stimulated lymphocytes plus IL2 was used for treatment of intraperitoneal Renca cell tumour [37]. Administration of chemoimmunotherapy into the peritoneal cavity resulted in cures of 90% of the tumour-bearing mice. Based on such encouraging results, attempts were made to treat this transplantable tumour at a more ad-

vanced stage of disease, beginning at 3 weeks after tumour inoculation under the kidney capsule, when visible peritoneal and systemic metastases were already present. It was possible to achieve cures in up to 80% of tumour-bearing mice by chemoimmunotherapy, but only when the treatment was administered by both the intraperitoneal and intravenous routes [38]. In addition, removal of the tumour-bearing kidney was required for effective therapy. Such impressive results with advanced disease are quite encouraging and suggest that maximal reduction of tumour burden, by surgery and chemotherapy, as well as administration of immunotherapy into the regions of metastases, may be required for complete elimination of advanced metastatic tumours.

Therapy with Purified IL2-Activated NK Cells

The extensive preclinical data and also clinical observations indicate that adoptive immunotherapy with IL2-stimulated lymphocytes plus IL2 can induce substantial antitumour effects, even when treatment is initiated after metastases are established. However, there are several major problems with the current generation of therapeutic protocols. Most of the therapeutic effects have been partial and transient, the processing of the cells for therapy is very expensive and labour-intensive, and the high doses utilised for treatment have been associated with serious toxic side effects. It therefore will be important to carefully investigate the many parameters involved in this therapeutic approach to attempt to develop more effective and simpler therapeutic strategies.

It seems important to consider seriously whether the rather cumbersome process of harvesting large numbers of lymphocytes, culturing them in the presence of IL2, and then reinfusing them is indeed necessary, or whether it might be possible to reproduce the same effects *in vivo* by administration of IL2 alone. Administration of high doses of recombinant IL2 has been shown to induce substantial proliferation of lymphocytes *in vivo* [33,39-40]. As discussed above, high doses of recombinant IL2 alone have been therapeutically effective in some situations in the mouse therapy experiments, and some clinical responses have been observed in trials with IL2 alone [e.g., 41,42]. It is of interest that the clinical responses to IL2 alone have tended to occur in the same tumour types as those found to be responsive to therapy with LAK cells plus IL2. It would seem that if the optimal dose, schedule and route of administration of IL2 could be found for expansion of the relevant lymphocytes *in vivo*, it might be possible to obviate the need for the more cumbersome *in vitro* stimulation and expansion of effector cells, and adoptive transfer, to achieve therapeutic results. However, the optimal dose and schedule for recombinant IL2 is not yet known, especially with regard to clinical studies. Until the full potential of IL2 alone is known or realised, it seems very desirable to continue the major efforts with adoptive therapy, in which the effector cells can be more directly manipulated. A fundamental limitation to therapy by IL2 administration *in vivo* may be the inability to achieve sufficiently selective expansion of the desired effector cells. In contrast, *in vitro*, one has the ability to separate and highly purify the desired effector cells and to remove undesired suppressive or inhibitory factors that may strongly interfere with the generation of high levels of effector-cell activity. It is also unclear whether it will be possible to achieve the desired optimal *in vivo* expansion of effector cells by the administration of IL2 alone, without incurring serious toxic side effects. In some circumstances, it appears that this should be possible. For example, Riccardi et al. [43] observed that rather low doses of IL2 were able to substantially stimulate the generation of NK cells from bone-marrow precursors in chimaeric mice. Also, Talmadge et al. [44] observed that quite low doses of IL2 as well as much higher doses of IL2 could have therapeutic effects in T cell-competent mice. Administration into the region of tumour growth may be a useful strategy to more selectively expand effector cells in the region of the tumour without inducing severe systemic toxic reactions. The number of effector cells actually required for therapeutic effects is not clear. The adoptive therapy studies performed to date have utilised unfractionated mononuclear cells. It

may be possible to achieve a substantially more favourable situation if effector cells are first isolated and purified. This should substantially decrease the requirement for the total number of cells and may also help to eliminate suppressor cells as well as irrelevant T cells. This might also substantially alter the requirement for IL2, since the dose needed to stimulate and expand a relatively small number of cells might be considerably less than that required for effects on a much larger number of total responding lymphocytes.

Recently, a new and simple procedure for the purification and rapid expansion of LAK cells from peripheral blood and splenic LGL has been developed [45]. This procedure exploits the observation made in our laboratory that rat LGL/NK cells initially respond to IL2 by adhering to plastic surfaces. As short as 2 hours after the addition of IL2, LGL adhere to plastic. This adherence is maximal at 24 to 48 hours in culture. These adherent cells are 94-97% LGL and express surface markers characteristic of rat NK cells, including OX8, asialo GM_1 and laminin. The cells did not express pan T cell (CD5), helper T cell (CD4) or B cell (Ig) markers, nor did they express the rat T cell-associated IL2 receptor, OX39. While 2-hour adherent cells show high levels of cytotoxic activity against YAC-1 targets only (NK activity), 48-hour adherent cells already demonstrate the development of high levels of LAK activity. The adherent LGL cells exhibiting LAK activity have been designated A-LAK cells.

When 48-hour A-LAK cells were separated from the non-adherent cells, washed and re-fed with conditioned medium, they rapidly expanded over the next 3 to 4 days, with expansion indices often reaching 90-fold in this time period. These expanding cells generated very high levels of cytotoxic LAK activity. When compared to the levels of cytotoxic LAK activity generated in standard bulk cultures, the adherent cultures generated between 20 and 50 times more total lytic units per culture. Studies of the phenotype of the rat A-LAK cells after expansion for 5 days or more in culture indicated that these cells are LGL and express surface markers (CD5) or helper T cell (CD4) markers and do not express significant levels of rat IL2 receptor (Tac type), as detected by the OX39 MoAb. These activated lymphocytes display cytolytic activity against neoplastic cells from a wide variety of tumours. Cytolytic activity could be demonstrated against tumour lines from different tissues and cell preparations, including ascites tumours, solid tumours, or neoplastic cell lines grown *in vitro* or *in vivo*.

In a series of studies, A-LAK cells have been utilised for therapy of experimental animal tumours, in both rats [46] and mice (Gorelik and Gunji, unpublished observations). The initial results of these studies have been highly encouraging, indicating that the purified A-LAK cells have substantially stronger anti-metastatic effects than unpurified LAK cells obtained by culturing mononuclear cells in the presence of IL2. Utilising the MCA-105 sarcoma in BALB/c mice, the same metastatic tumour model used by Rosenberg and his colleagues for most of their experimental therapy studies, A-LAK cells gave strong antimetastatic effects at cell numbers considerably below those needed to produce significant effects with standard LAK cells. With the B16/BL6 melanoma, a mouse tumour that is quite resistant to therapeutic effects of standard LAK cells, relatively low numbers of purified A-LAK cells produced considerable reduction in lung metastases, when administered with a modest dose of IL2. Strong therapeutic effects with A-LAK cells have also been seen with a rat experimental breast cancer, MADB106 [46]. Even when the same total amount of *in vitro* measured cytotoxic activity (i.e., same total lytic units) was transferred to the recipient tumour-bearing rats, the purified effector cells were considerably more active therapeutically, against both pulmonary and hepatic metastases, than standard, unpurified LAK cells.

Mechanism of Anti-Tumour Therapeutic Effects of Adoptively Transferred Effector Cells

In addition to the expected value of purified cells for use in therapy, the availability of more defined cell populations permits more detailed examination of the mechanism by which such cells might mediate their therapeutic effects. The first issue to be considered is the *in vivo* distribution of the adoptively transferred cells. One would predict that therapeutic effects would be dependent on these cells reaching the tumour site or at least accumulating in the vicinity of the tumour. Although *in vivo* distribution of LAK cells, prepared in the usual manner, has previously been examined, interpretation of the results with such unpurified, heterogeneous cell populations is fraught with difficulty. The concern is that the *in vivo* distribution information would mainly reflect the distribution of the predominant cell type in the population rather than that of the effector cells. Furthermore, if uptake of some transferred cells were demonstrated in the tumour lesions, it would be unclear which cells were represented and whether they included cells with antitumour effector function. Based on such considerations, my laboratory has been utilising A-LAK cells to study the *in vivo* distribution of these defined cells with therapeutic potential.

Our initial studies were performed with a radiolabel as a marker for the distribution of the cells *in vivo*. Studies performed with ^{51}Cr-labelled rat A-LAK cells revealed initial uptake of most of the label in the lungs after intravenous inoculation, followed by redistribution mainly to the liver and the spleen by 24 hours [47]. In contrast to T cells, A-LAK cells showed no ability to accumulate in lymph nodes [48]. More recent studies have indicated that ^{51}Cr as a cellular label may provide an overestimate of uptake of cells in the liver, presumably by accumulation of released free metal, and that ^{125}IUdR is a more reliable indicator of *in vivo* distribution (P. Basse, R.B. Herberman and R.H. Goldfarb, unpublished observations). However, with either label, there has been little indication of a significant uptake of labelled cells in primary or metastatic tumours, above that measured in normal tissues or in the same organ uninvolved by tumour. We considered the possibility that failure to detect significant accumulation of effector cells in tumours, especially in tumour models showing therapeutic effects by the transferred cells, might be due to insufficient sensitivity of the radioisotopic technique. If there were accumulation of only small numbers of effector cells at the tumour site, the levels of associated radioactivity might not be detectable above background levels.

To explore this issue, we have utilised fluorescent dyes to label mouse A-LAK cells and have studied their distribution in mice with experimental metastases induced by the B16F1 melanoma. Intravenous inoculation of tumour cells induces experimental pulmonary metastases and liver metastases can be induced by left ventricular inoculation of a liver-homing variant of B16F1 cells. After intravenous inoculation of fluorescent A-LAK cells, at one hour the uptake of cells in normal lungs was similar to that detectable in tumour-bearing mice (P. Basse, R.B. Herberman and R.H. Goldfarb, manuscript in preparation). At this time point, there was no indication of selective uptake by tumour metastases; however, by 16-18 hours there appeared to be a redistribution of cells within the lungs of tumour-bearing mice, with an average of 20-fold greater localisation in pulmonary metastases relative to normal lung tissue. However, very few cells per metastasis were observed, with some metastases showing no detectable uptake of the transferred cells. After intraarterial inoculation, there was increased uptake of fluorescent cells in other major organs, including the liver. After intraportal inoculation, there was much higher uptake in the liver and a substantial proportion of metastases contained fluorescent A-LAK cells (P. Basse, R.B. Herberman and R.H. Goldfarb, manuscript in preparation).

The failure of transferred cells to appreciably accumulate in the metastases may account for the only partial therapeutic efficacy that has been observed for adoptive immunotherapy with A-LAK cells in this B16 tumour model. However, a further major question raised by these results is how might the small number of effector cells that accumulate in at least some of the tumour lesions result in complete regression of some metastases. Although one might have expected that *in vivo* therapeutic results might be due to direct cytotoxicity, as measured with the effector cells *in vitro*, this seems quite unlikely since the apparent effector:target cell ratios in the experimental metastases were very low, usually less than 1:1. An alternative explanation for therapeutic efficacy might be local cytokine production by the A-LAK cells. A-LAK cells have been shown to produce substantial levels of TNF-alpha and interferon gamma. Perhaps small numbers of cells at the tumour site could secrete sufficient amounts of these and possibly other factors to amplify their effects and to enlist the involvement of other effector cells. Consistent with this possibility has been the observation that A-LAK cells (mouse and rat) produce a variety of proteolytic enzymes, similar to those that are associated with the invasive properties of metastatic tumour cells, for penetration of basement membranes (R.H. Goldfarb, R.P. Kitson and R.B. Herberman, manuscript in preparation).

One major unanswered question, which is quite relevant to the above considerations, is whether the adoptively transferred cells are able to emigrate out of the microvasculature into tumour tissues and then directly interact with tumour cells. To examine this issue, we have recently utilised a novel animal model that permits visualisation of the microvasculature of normal and tumour-bearing tissues [49]. These studies have involved vital video microscopy of the microvasculature of chambers in the ears of rabbits, containing granulation tissue or the VX2 carcinoma, a transplantable rabbit tumour that induces extensive neovascularisation. Human A-LAK cells have been inoculated into the artery of the ear of normal or tumour-bearing rabbits. As in the studies of A-LAK cell distribution in mice, only a very small proportion of the inoculated cells were retained in the microvasculature of either normal or tumour-bearing ears. However, it was possible to observe selective and longer retention of transferred A-LAK cells in the tumour microvasculature, and this retention appeared to be confined to adherence in the post-capillary venules. Over a period of observation of up to 24 hours, there was no indication that these cells retained in the microvasculature emigrated into the tumour tissues. Despite this apparent failure of the transferred cells to directly interact with tumour cells, focal necrosis of tumours has been observed to occur in this model system. Histologic sections of treated tumours at about one week after inoculation showed not only evidence of necrosis, but also substantial accumulation of a variety of inflammatory cells, including macrophages and eosinophils in addition to lymphocytes.

These recent results indicate involvement of a novel mechanism for the therapeutic effects, which had not been previously considered. From this study as well as from the studies with mouse tumour cells, direct cytotoxic effects seem unlikely to account for the therapeutic efficacy that has been observed. Production of cytokines by a small number of effector cells seems to be a real possibility, but this would appear to occur at some distance from the tumour cells. In addition to the possibility of cytokines directly inhibiting the growth of tumour cells, the haemostasis and focal necrosis seen in the rabbit ear model strongly suggest that the antitumour effects may be indirect via changes in the microvasculature. It is intriguing to consider the possibility that one or a few A-LAK cells might have major effects after attaching to the tumour microvasculature, perhaps by secreting cytokines like TNF that might induce attachment of granulocytes to endothelial cells and also induce coagulation, or the attached effector cells might damage or activate the endothelial cells, with this in turn leading to the observed changes. Further studies are needed to distinguish among these possibilities and also to determine the basis for the selective retention of A-LAK cells in the post capillary venules of the tumour microvasculature. Insights into these and related issues may help to understand the basis for therapeutic efficacy and allow the rational development of improved strategies for adoptive cellular therapy.

REFERENCES

1 Yamada S, Ruscetti FW, Overton WR, Herberman RB and Ortaldo JR: Regulation of human large granular lymphocytes and T cell growth and function by recombinant interleukin 2. I. Induction of interleukin 2 receptor and promotion of growth of cells with enhanced cytotoxicity. J Leuk Biol 1987 (41):505-517

2 Bonnard GD, Yasaka K and Jacobson D: Ligand-activated T cell growth factor-induced T-cell proliferation. Absorption of T cell growth factor by activated T cells. J Immun 1979 (123):2704-2708

3 Talmadge JE, Wiltrout RH, Counts DF, Herberman RB, McDonald T and Ortaldo JR: Proliferation of human peripheral blood lymphocytes induced by recombinant human interleukin-2: Contribution of large granular lymphocytes and T lymphocytes. Cell Immunol 1986 (102):261-272

4 Ortaldo JR, Mason AT, Gerard JP, Henderson LE, Farrar W, Hopkins RF III, Herberman RB, and Rabin H: Effects of natural and recombinant IL-2 on regulation of IFN production and natural killer activity: Lack of involvement of the Tac antigen for these immunoregulatory effects. J Immun 1984 (133):779-783

5 Grimm EA, Mazumder A, Zhang HZ and Rosenberg SA: Lymphokine-activated killer cell phenomenon, lysis of natural killer cell resistant fresh solid tumor cells by interleukin-2-activated autologous human peripheral blood lymphocytes. J Exp Med 1982 (155):823-830

6 Grimm EA, Ramsey KM, Mazumder A, Wilson DJ, Djeu JY and Rosenberg SA: Lymphokine activated killer cell phenomenon. II. Precursor phenotype is serologically distinct from peripheral T lymphocytes, memory cytotoxic tymus-derived lymphocytes and natural killer cells. J Exp Med 1983 (157):884-897

7 Herberman RB, Balch C, Bolhuis R, Golub S, Hiserodt J, Lanier L, Lotzova E, Phillips J, Riccardi C, Ritz J, Santoni A, Schmidt R, Uchida A, and Vujanovic N: Lymphokine-activated killer cell activity: characteristics of effector cells and their progenitors in blood and spleen. Immunol Today 1987 (8):178-181

8 Rosenberg EB, Herberman RB, Levine PH, Halterman RH, McCoy JL and Wunderlich JR: Lymphocyte cytotoxicity reactions to leukemia-associated antigens in identical twins. Int J Cancer 1972 (9):648-658

9 McCoy JL, Herberman RB, Rosenberg EB, Donnelly FC, Levine PH and Alford C: 51Chromium release assay for cell-mediated cytotoxicity of human leukemia and lymphoid tissue-culture cells. NCI Monogr 1973 (37):59-67

10 Rosenberg EB, McCoy JL, Green SS, Donnelly FC, Siwarski DF, Levine PH and Herberman RB: Destruction of human lymphoid tissue culture cell lines by human peripheral lymphocytes in 51Cr-release cellular cytotoxicity assays. JNCI 1974 (52):345-352

11 Gorelik E, Wiltrout R, Okumura K, Habu S and Herberman R: Role of NK cells in the control of metastatic spread and growth of tumor cells in mice. Int J Cancer 1982 (30):107

12 Barlozzari T, Reynolds C and Herberman R: In vivo role of natural killer cells: involvement of large granular lymphocytes in the clearance of tumor cells in anti-asailo GM1-treated rats. J Immun 1983 (131):1024

13 Barlozzari T, Leonhardt J, Wiltrout R, Herberman R and Reynolds C: Direct evidence for the role of LGL in the inhibition of experimental tumor metastases. J Immun 1985 (134):2783-2789

14 Uchida A and Micksche M: Lysis of fresh human tumor cells by autologous peripheral blood lymphocytes and pleural effusion lymphocytes activated by OK432. JNCI 1983 (71):673-680

15 Uchida A and Yanagawa E: Natural killer cell activity and autologous tumor killing activity in cancer patients: Overlapping involvement of effector cells as determined in two-target conjugate cytotoxicity assay. JNCI 1984 (73):1093-1100

16 Lotzova E Savary CA, Herberman RB and Dicke KA: Brief research news: Can NK cells play a role in therapy of leukemia?. Natural Immunity and Cell Growth Regulation 1986 (5):61-63

17 Lotzova E, Savary CA and Herberman RB: Induction of NK cell activity against fresh human leukemia in culture with interleukin-2. J Immun 1987 (138):2718-2727

18 DeVries R and Golub S: Target recognition by human NK cells and lymphokine activated killer cells. Feder Proc 1986 (45):a2760

19 Shau H and Golub SH: Depletion of NK cells with the lysosomotropic agent L-leucine methyl ester and the in vitro generation of NK activity from NK precursor cells. J Immun 1985 (134):1136-1141

20 Hercend T, Meuer SC, Brennan A, Edson MA, Acuto O, Reinherz EL, Schlossman SF, and Ritz J: Identification of a clonally restricted 90 KD heterodimer on two cloned natural killer cell lines: Its role in cytotoxic effector function. J Exp Med 1983 (158):1547-1560

21 Schmidt RE, Hercend T, Fox DA, Bewnsussan A, Bartley G, Daley JF, Schlossman SF, Reinherz EL and Ritz J: The role of interleukin-2 and T11-E rosette antigen in activation and proliferation of human NK clones. J Immun 1985 (135):672-678

22 Damle NK, Doyle LV and Bradley EC: Interleukin-2-activated human killer cells are derived from phenotypically heterogeneous precursors. J Immun 1986 (137):2814-2822

23 Reynolds CW, Sharrow SO, Ortaldo JR and Herberman RB: Natural killer activity in the rat. III. Analysis of surface antigens on LGL by flow cytometry. J Immun 1981 (127):2204

24 Hiserodt JC, Laybourn KA and Varani J: Expression of a laminin-like substance on the surface of murine natural killer (NK) lymphocytes and its role in NK recognition of tumor target cells. J Immun 1985 (135):1481

25 Vujanovic NL, Herberman RB, Olszowy MW, Cramer DV, Salup RR, Reynolds CW and Hiserodt JC: Lymphokine-activated killer cells in rats: analysis of progenitor and effector cell phenotype and relationship to natural killer cells. Cancer Res 1988 (48):884-890

26 Gunji Y, Vujanovic NL, Hiserodt JC, Herberman RB and Gorelik E: Generation and characterization of purified adherent lymphokine-activated killer cells in mice. J Immun 1989 (142):1748-1754

27 Shortman K, Wilson A and Scollay R: Loss of specificity in cytolytic T lymphocyte clones obtained by limit dilution culture of Lyt-2+ T cells. J Immun 1984 (132):584-593

28 Hercend T, Reinherz EL, Meuer SC, Schlossman SF and Ritz J: Phenotypic and functional heterogeneity of human cloned natural killer cell lines. Nature 1983 (30):158-160

29 Van de Griend RJ, Giphart MJ, Van Krimpen BA, Bolhuis RL: Human T cell clones exerting multiple cytolytic activities show heterogeneity in susceptibility to inhibition by monoclonal antibodies. J Immun 1984 (133):1222-1229

30 Kedar E, Ikejiri BL, Gorelik E and Herberman RB: Natural cell-mediated cytotoxicity in vitro and inhibition of tumor growth in vivo by murine lymphoid cells cultured with T cell growth factor (TCGF). Clin Immunol Immunother 1982 (13):14-23

31 Mule JJ, Shu S, Schwarz SL and Rosenberg SA: Adoptive immunotherapy of established pulmonary metastases with LAK cells and recombinant interleukin-2. Science 1984 (225):1487-1489

32 Mule JJ, Shu S and Rosenberg SA: The anti-tumor efficacy of lymphokine-activated killer cells and recombinant interleukin 2 in vivo. J Immun 1985 (135):646-652

33 Ettinghausen SE, Lipford EH, Mule JJ and Rosenberg SA: Systemic administration of recombinant interleukin 2 stimulates in vivo lymphoid cell proliferation in tissues. J Immun 1985 (135):1488-1497

34 Ettinghausen SE, Lipford EH, Mule JJ and Rosenberg SA: Recombinant interleukin 2 stimulates in vivo proliferation of adaptively transferred lymphokine-activated killer (LAK) cells. J Immun 1985 (135):3623-3635

35 Salup RR and Wiltrout RH: Adjuvant immunotherapy of established murine renal cancer by interleukin 2-stimulated cytotoxic lymphocytes. Cancer Res 1986 (46):3358-3363

36 Rosenberg SA, Lotze MT, Muul LM, Leitman S, Chang AE, Ettinghausen SE, Matory YL, Skibber JM, Shiloni E, Vetto JT et al: Observations on the systemic administration of autologous lymphokine-activated killer cells and recombinant interleukin-2 to patients with metastatic cancer. N Engl J Med 1985 (313):1485-1492

37 Salup RR and Wiltrout RH: Treatment of adenocarcinoma in the peritoneum of mice: chemoimmunotherapy with IL-2-stimulated cytotoxic lymphocytes as a model for treatment of minimal residual disease. Cancer Immunol Immunother 1986 (22):31-36

38 Salup RR and Wiltrout RH: Successful treatment of advanced murine renal cancer by bicompartmental administration of adoptive chemoimmunotherapy. J Immun 1987 (138):641-647

39 Cheever MA, Thompson JA, Kern DE and Greenberg PD: Interleukin 2 (IL2) administred in vivo: influence of IL-2 route and timing on T cell growth. J Immun 1985 (134):3895-3900

40 Lotze MT, Matory YL, Ettinghausen SE, Reyner AA, Sharrow SO, Seipp CA, Custer MC and Rosenberg SA: In vivo administration of purified human interleukin 2. II. Half life, immunologic effects, and expansion of peripheral lymphoid cells in vivo with recombinant IL2. J Immun 1985 (135):2865-2875

41 Rosenberg SA, Lotze MT, Muul LM, Chang AE, Avis FP, Leitman S, Linehan WM, Robertson CN, Lee RE, Rubin JT, Seipp CA, Simpson CG and White DE: Progress report on the treatment of 157 patients with advanced cancer using lymphokine-activated killer cells and interleukin-2 or high-dose interleukin-2 alone. N Engl J Med 1987 (316):889-897

42 West WH, Taver KW, Yannelli JR, Marshall GD, Orr DW, Thurman GB and Oldham RK: Constant-infusion recombinant interleukin-2 in adoptive immunotherapy of advanced cancer. N Engl J Med 1987 (316):898-905

43 Riccardi C, Giampietri A, Migliorati G, Cannarile L, D'Adamio L and Herberman RB: Generation of mouse natural killer (NK) cell activity: effect of interleukin-2 (IL2) and interferon (IFN) on the in vivo development of natural killer cells from bone marrow (BM) progenitor cells. Int J Cancer 1986 (38):553-562

44 Talmadge JE, Phillips H, Schindler J, Tribble H and Pennington R: Systematic preclinical study on the therapeutic properties of recombinant human interleukin 2 for the treatment of metastatic disease. Cancer Res 1987 (47):5725-5732

45 Vujanovic NL, Herberman RB, Al Maghazachi A and Hiserodt JC: Lymphokine-activated killer cells in rats. III. A simple method for the purification of large granular lymphocytes and their rapid expansion and conversion into lymphokine activated killer cells. J Exp Med 1988 (267):15-29

46 Schwarz RE, Vujanovic NL and Hiserodt JC: Enhanced antimetastatic activity of lymphokine-activated killer cells purified and expanded by their adherence to plastic. Cancer Res 1989 (49):1441-1446

47 Al Maghazachi A, Herberman RB, Vujanovic NL and Hiserodt, JC: In vivo distribution and tissue localization of highly purified rat lymphokine ctivated killer (LAK) cells. Cell Immunol 1988 (115):179-194

48 Al Maghazachi A, Goldfarb RH and Herberman RB: Influence of T cells on the expression of lymphokine-activated killer cell activity and in vivo tissue distribution. J Immun 1988 (141):4039-4046

49 Sasaki A, Melder RJ, Jain RK, Whiteside TL and Herberman RB: Preferential localization of human adherent lymphokine-activated killer (A-LAK) cells in tumor microcirculation: a novel mechanism for adoptive immunotherapy. Submitted for publication

Interleukin 2: In Vivo Induction of Effector Cells

Guido Forni [1], Maria Carla Bosco [2], Stefania Vai [2] and Mirella Giovarelli [3]

1   Centro di Immunogenetica ed Istocompatibilita', CNR, Turin, Italy
2   Institute of Microbiology, University of Turin, Turin, Italy
3   Department of Experimental Medicine, University of L'Aquila, L'Aquila, Italy

The immune system possesses distinct effector mechanisms that destroy not-self as well as self-altered cells. Their power is so high that the system devotes great care to their induction, coordination and modulation. The intricacy of regulatory manoeuvres is thus a dominant feature of the immune system [1]. Complex cell-cell communications are required to govern multicellular events. One cell communication code is made by the network of receptor idiotypes [2]. A second depends on the expression of nonspecific adhesion-receptor molecules that allow the establishment of defined cell-cell contacts. A further code is based on the polymorphism of the membrane glycoproteins coded by the major histocompatibility complex (MHC). Their selective expression and ability to bind foreign and own peptides, and to interact with the T-lymphocyte receptor (TCR), are the basis for the induction of specific responses [3].

Interleukins (ILs) belong to another communication code of the immune system. Of these, IL2 is in many ways a prototype. Activation of the IL2 gene, transduction of IL2 mRNA, secretion of IL2 molecules and their autocrine or paracrine interaction with the multi-chain membrane receptors, are key events during the evolution of a cell-mediated immune response. This explains why the IL2 and IL2 receptor system are probably best characterised of the ILs in terms of both molecular biochemistry and function [4].

Comprehension of the IL code is of paramount importance, since it allows one to understand a few of the rules that govern immune reactions. Moreover, by using the constituents of this code it could be possible to manipulate natural events with some degree of precision. In effect, the progressive availability of ILs and their agonists and antagonists provided by recombinant DNA technology could open the way to regulation of many features of the immune response [5].

This possibility is particularly appealing in tumour immunology. In many *in vitro* systems, as well as in *in vivo* preimmunisation experiments, the immune system has been shown to be potentially capable of inhibiting autochthonous or syngeneic tumour growth. By contrast, however, most spontaneous or transplanted tumours grow and kill their host. This paradoxical hallmark of host-tumour immune relationship could be cancelled by the pharmacological addition of regulatory ILs. In this dynamic relationship, the early outcome of tumour-borne negative interferences with regulatory mechanisms of the immune system is a feature of critical importance, on which both the poor immunogenicity of tumours and the ease with which they induce suppression often depend [5,6].

The current challenge is to learn how to use IL2 and other ILs to make meaningful messages able to guide an anti-tumour response in tumour-bearing hosts.

How IL2 Works During an Immune Response

To achieve this goal, a few characteristics of the IL2 system must be taken into account (Table 1) [4,7-8]. IL2 is an inducible glycopro-

Table 1. A few characteristics of the human IL2 system

The IL2 molecule

---

* 15 kD glycoproteins of 133 amino acids organised in 6 α-helix barrels and small interconnecting random-coil regions

* Coded by a single autosomal gene pair on chromosome 4q (4 exons)

* Its conformational structure is essential for the interaction with cell membrane receptors.

* Half-life in serum: minutes

The IL2 receptor complex *

	p55 (Tac,CD25)	p75	p55+p75
Molecular weight (kD)	55-45	75	55+75
Affinity constant (Kd nM)	10	1	0.01
T 1/2 association	5 sec	45 min	30 sec
T 1/2 dissociation	7 sec	300 min	280 min
Internalisation	no	yes	yes
Shedding	50, 45 Kd	no	no
Biological activity	? soluble	yes	yes
Sites/cell	25-50,000	2-4,000	2-4,000
Signal transduction	no (?)	yes	yes
Expression by quiescent leukocytes	no	>90% NK,<5% B,T macrophages	-
Inducibility on partially activated leukocytes	yes	macrophages, other ?	yes

* [4,5,7-9]

tein mainly secreted by activated T lymphocytes and NK cells. The human IL2 gene has been cloned and production of recombinant (r), not glycosylated IL2 by transfected Escherichia coli has become possible. Once secreted, IL2 may interact with nearby cell membrane receptors formed by at least 2 distinct molecules.

One (p75) is constitutively expressed by a small proportion of peripheral blood lymphocytes (5-15%, depending on the donor), embracing all CD16+ cells, less than 5% of B and T lymphocytes, and neither resting monocytes nor granulocytes [4,5,7,8]. p75 binds IL2 with intermediate affinity and transduces the signal into the cell. Then its expression starts to be down-regulated.

A second receptor molecule (p55, Tac antigen or CD25) binds IL2 with low affinity and apparently does not transduce the signal into the cell. It is not expressed by resting leukocytes but appears on the membranes of T and B lymphocytes, monocytes and endothelial cells following initial cell activation [4,8].

About 5% of the p55 molecules on the cell membrane interact via noncovalent forces with the p75 chain to create a heterodimeric p55-p75 receptor that binds IL2 with very high affinity. p55 molecules are shed in the form of p50 and p45 soluble fragments.

The gradual binding of IL2, secreted by the same lymphocyte (autocrinally) or by a nearby one (paracrinally or in a polarised way), to either receptor builds up a threshold that allows the progression of lymphocyte activation. It makes T lymphocytes pass from the G to the S phase of the cell cycle and activates the c-myb gene [4].

The 4 main variables that control IL2 activity in a quantal manner are: a) the number of receptors on the cell membrane; b) the IL2 concentration in the environment; c) the time of interaction between IL2 and its receptor; d) the kind of receptor expressed by target cells [4]. Paracrinally secreted IL2 or IL2 present in the cell culture medium is thus a nonspecific signal that acts on any cell then expressing an IL2 receptor. The IL2 signal acquires selectivity or even specificity via 3 mechanisms: a) modulation of membrane expression of p75, p55 and p55-p75 receptors; b) very short IL2 half-life (minutes) in body fluids; c) manner of IL2 secretion [4,9,10].

Receptors that have bound IL2 are taken into the cell. Circulating IL2 is mostly degraded by the kidney. The presence of serum inhibitors and the intense shedding of p55 receptors following lymphocyte activation may also provide local inhibition. These clearance systems make IL2 evanescent and prevent it, when secreted in a micro site of the immune system, from exercising widespread effects. As a result, IL2 does not behave as an hormone of the immune system, but rather as a cell-cell transmitter [3-5].

On many occasions, 2 lymphocytes gather to deliver or receive an IL2 message. In this case, the cell-cell contacting phase is specific: first, the lymphocytes recognise selective adhesion molecules, then TCR specifically interacts with MHC glycoproteins bound to foreign peptides. Once the conjugate is formed, a polarised secretion of IL2 as well as other ILs takes place primarily over the small area of cell-cell contact. In this way, the specificity of the message is maintained (Fig.1A) [3,10]. Paracrine IL2 secretion may also take place in spleen or lymph nodes, where the secreted

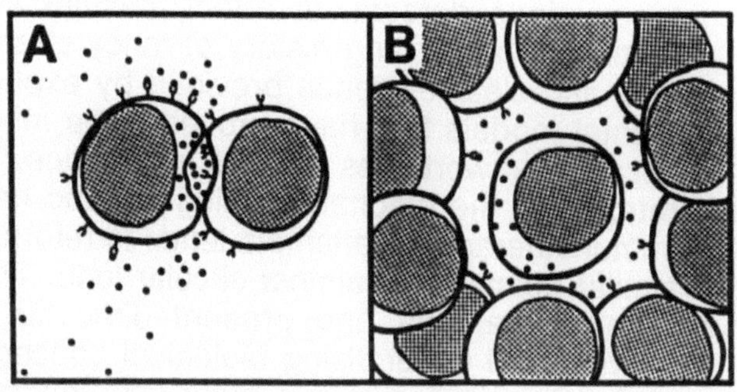

Fig. 1. Modes of IL2 secretion.
Panel A: An IL2 secreting (helper) lymphocyte (left) contacts a partner cell in an antigen-restricted or nonspecific way. When the conjugate is formed, a polarised secretion of IL2 as well as other lymphokines takes place primarily in the area of cell contacts. The same helper lymphocyte can autocrinally utilise the lymphokines secreted in order to progress in the cell cycle.
Panel B: Paracrine IL2 secretion can also take place in spleen or lymph nodes. An IL2 secreting cell can lead to the activation of leukocytes packed around the helper cell

IL2 is not diluted too quickly. In this way, an IL2-secreting lymphocyte can recruit various kinds of tightly packed nearby cells (Fig.1B). Here, the selectivity of the IL2 paracrine delivery depends on the type of IL2 receptor expressed by resting or activated nearby lymphocytes and on the amount of IL2 secreted, since its efficiency decreases as the distance between the cells increases. Secreted IL2 can also be autocrinally utilised by the same cell to progress in the cell cycle (Fig.1A). Even if autocrine IL2 utilisation seems to be a common feature of T-lymphocyte activation, it is difficult to assess its significance *in vivo* because of quick IL2 flushing, inhibition by body fluids, and competitive absorption by nearby cells [9].

Killer Strategies: Concepts and Findings

If the scenario described above is basically correct, what kind of strategies can be envisaged for IL2 use in tumour immunotherapy? The unlimited availability of rIL2 has made it possible to hark back to old and unsuccessful battle plans and try to wipe out the memory of ignominious defeats. In effect, cellular immunology has a long history of fancy strategies and clear evidence provided by experimental models that have proved to be inapplicable or worthless in clinical practice. In retrospect, the rationale guiding old and new immunotherapeutic attempts tends to return to similar points in an almost circular loop. This reflects the past and present difficulty of proving and generalising biological concepts underlying strategies in tumour immunotherapy [9,11]. A large series of studies has suggested that cytotoxic T lymphocytes (CTL) recognising tumour-associated antigens (TAA) in association with MHC glycoproteins can afford protection against authochthonous and syngeneic tumours [12]. When IL2 was first characterised as a T-cell growth factor, it appeared capable of overcoming the difficulty of obtaining large quantities of specifically reactive CTL or CTL clones. These expanded populations maintain their ability to kill tumour cells when injected *in vivo*, and their survival can be prolonged by repeated administration of low doses of IL2 [12-14]. A few practical problems hindered this approach. CTLs are chiefly active in immunosuppressed hosts, their activity can be impaired by self- or tumour-elicited specific suppression, and only a few of them are still able to reach the tumour mass [12,15-16]. Overall, this specific approach rests on the assumption that tumour cells express TAAs that can be recognised by CTLs.

The progressively growing belief that human tumours are not immunogenic [17,18] strongly limited the development of this approach and diverted much interest from specific immunotherapy to the exploitation of NK cell activity. NK cells do not recognise TAA, but rather more widespread structures on susceptible target cell membranes. Substantial evidence points to their involvement in immunosurveillance against primary tumours and blood-borne metastases in particular [18]. It was also found that their activity is characteristically boosted by interferons (IFN) and IL2. However, multiple treatments with agents able to enhance NK cytotoxicity eventually result in reduced or undetectable augmentation of NK activity. A major challenge still remains to determine how to obtain prolonged augmentation of NK activity and whether this will result in a more effective control of tumour growth [19].

While these difficulties made clinical exploitation of cellular reactivity against cancer remote, the discovery by E. Grimm et al., of lymphokine-activated killer (LAK) activity [20] appeared to be an important new finding. The incubation of fresh peripheral blood lymphocytes (PBL) with 1,000 units of IL2 for 3-5 days results in their acquisition of a strong lytic activity against a large variety of fresh tumour cells, including those which are NK resistant, while sparing most normal tissues. In the initial papers, LAK activity was attributed to a new leukocyte lineage. By contrast, an overwelming number of experimental data have shown that it is mostly induced on the 5-15% PBL that constitutively expresses the p75 IL2 receptor on the cell membrane (almost all CD16+ CD3- NK and only <5% of T- and B-lymphocytes) [21,22].

The discovery of LAK activity, distinct from NK and CTL lytic functions, opened fresh approaches to cancer immunotherapy. In a variety of experimental mouse-tumour models, the intravenous adoptive transfer of LAK cells generated *in vitro*, in conjunction with repeated injections of high doses of rIL2, caused the regression of established pulmonary metastases [23,24]. Following this line, a paper by Rosenberg et al. [25] in December 1985 reported the first clinical results of a protocol based on the repeated administration of human LAK cells in combination with IL2 in patients with advanced cancer. As this seminal protocol, its clinical outcome and its numerous developments and repeats are discussed in other sections of this monograph, only general biological considerations will be put forward here.

The main problem stems from the fact that the immune system utilises IL2 as a quickly absorbed, inhibited and catabolised cell-cell transmitter, and not at all as a systemic immune hormone [26]. Therefore, impressive amounts of rIL2, close to the maximum tolerated doses, have to be repeatedly injected to maintain in the body fluids the pharmacological levels necessary to preserve LAK activity. The presence of such high levels of IL2 induces dramatic dose-related side effects in cancer patients that quickly disappear on suspension of the treatment [27]. These side effects appear to be a consequence of the

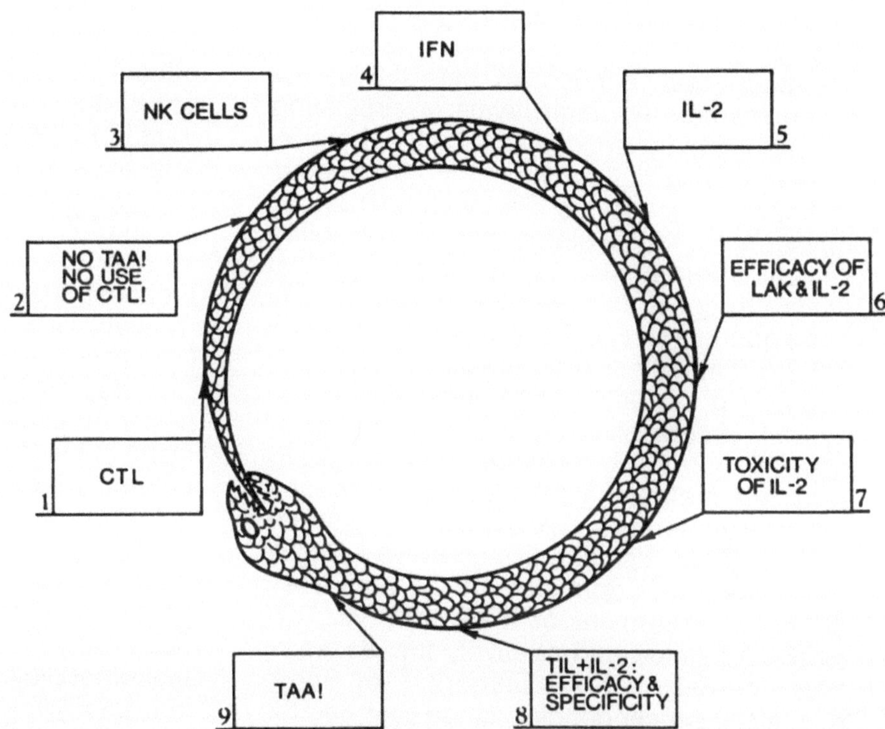

Fig. 2. Passage from specific to nonspecific tumor immunotherapy strategies: A circular path [11]

many activities turned on in host lymphoid cells by the high levels of circulating IL2. Moreover, it still remains to be shown whether these are only side-effects that must be eliminated, or if they play major role in LAK-cell mediated tumour lysis *in vivo* [27,28]. This question is related to another major - paradoxical - problem: are LAK cells an important component of the IL2-LAK immunotherapeutic regimen?

The original aim of maintaining elevated body fluid IL2 levels was to keep LAK cells fully active in the hostile environment of the tumour-bearing body. In effect, the basic idea and the most common interpretation of experimental and clinical findings were straightforward: PBLs cultured in the presence of rIL2 acquire LAK activity, i.e., efficiently kill fresh tumour cells *in vitro*. LAK cells can be adoptively transferred into mice or patients with tumours, where they kill tumour cells and determine tumour remissions, provided IL2 is continuously infused to sustain their activity. These concepts directly come from many studies on the passive transfer of cytotoxic cells and restrict the biological role of IL2 to a growth factor activity.

Nevertheless, other studies by Rosenberg's group have shown that high doses of rIL2 can act as a direct *in vivo* immunomodulator. In the mouse, high doses of rIL2 injected every 9 hours stimulate lymphoid cell proliferation in the tissues, enhance NK activity, induce LAK activity, increase the reactivity of previously generated CTL, and inhibit the growth of various metastases. Sublethal mouse irradiation before treatment abolishes these effects, showing that rIL2 does not affect tumour growth directly, but activates host immune reactivity, while a direct correlation has been found between tumour inhibition and LAK cell generation [29,30].

While a few mouse models have made it clear that IL2 alone is less effective than IL2 + LAK cells [23], clinical trials suggest that this may not be the case in man. This point has immediate practical interest, since, if rIL2 alone is active, the complex preparation of LAK cells and their passive transfer can be avoided. Several ongoing clinical trials with cancer patients are considering the systemic, regional or local use of rIL2 only. Some successes have been obtained (see other sections of this monograph). Indeed, if IL2 alone is fully active, or if the presence of LAK cells adds only a minor increase in anti-tumour efficacy, the rationale of LAK plus IL2 therapy is wrong.

Treatment with either LAK plus IL2 or IL2 alone requires the high levels of circulating IL2 associated with adverse effects. The possibility of using rIL2 to expand *in vitro* tumour infiltrating lymphocytes (TIL) was next tested in experimental systems and is attracting clinical interest [31,32]. In effect, several studies suggest that the non-immunogenicity of human tumours is more apparent than real [33-35]. TIL may also be present in a tumour because of a specific TAA recognition. The careful, progressive expansion in the presence of rIL2 of TIL recovered from surgically resected melanoma metastases or murine tumours generates a population of lymphocytes that can also express selective killing of the tumour cells from which they have been obtained. Treatment of mice with TIL, cyclophosphamide and relatively low doses of rIL2 mediates the elimination of large metastatic cancer deposits in the liver and the lungs more than 100 times more efficiently than conventional IL2 plus LAK cell therapy [31,32]. The therapeutic approaches based on TIL utilisation are promising. Low non-toxic doses of IL2 have to be used. Besides their higher ability to reach the tumour and cause its rapid regression, TIL may also establish a long-lasting immune memory. However, a semantic ambiguity is intrinsic in the IL2 activated TILs, which display variable degrees of both LAK and tumour-specific, CTL-type lytic activity. In this respect, TIL seems to conclude a purposeful immunological endeavour to inhibit neoplasia by the direct killing of tumour cells. The path both begins and ends with CTL (Fig. 2).

Direct Killing of Tumour Cells: What a Nonsense in Tumour Therapy!

In NK, LAK, TIL and CTL based immunotherapies, it is not obvious that the direct killing of tumour cells, as currently evaluated in *in vitro* tests, is the exact mechanism by which effector lymphocytes achieve their therapeutic effect *in vivo*. The *in vitro* training required to generate killer cells often results in a down-

modulation of their adhesion receptors that impairs their homing ability *in vivo*. On the other hand, the magnitude of the anti-tumour effects observed *in vivo* does not always correlate with the number of adoptively transferred killer lymphocytes present in the target tissue. This is so often evident with both CTL and LAK cells that it prevents a straight interpretation of the mechanisms responsible for their *in vivo* efficacy. Actually, it has been proposed that they may be nothing more than "helper" lymphocytes disguised as "killers" [19,11].

The data on the active role played by the systemic administration of high doses of IL2 alone show that even the immune system of a patient bearing a tumour can be effectively activated to mount such an efficient immune response that large tumour burdens are rapidly destroyed [36]. These high doses bypass the physiological control systems and IL2 behaves as a new kind of *in vivo* immunomodulator. In these conditions, IL2 both interacts with cells constitutively expressing the IL2 receptor inducing its up-modulation and turns on many effector mechanisms [4,25,29,30].

The IL2 pleiotropic activity, as detected *in vitro*, becomes even more evident *in vivo* because of the highly interactive nature of the immune system, where a signal delivered by an activated cell affects many others. Actually, the efficacy of IL2 *in vivo* may fully rest on the induction of this cascade of interconnected effector functions, each affecting neoplastic growth with distinct mechanisms and selectivity. The *in vitro* generated LAK cells, once passively transferred *in vivo*, may have an important killer role, but, by releasing multiple lymphokines, they may activate multiple host reaction mechanisms that play an even more substantial part in tumour inhibition [5].

Helper Strategies: All Together!

IL2 activated leukocytes thus assume both effector and regulatory functions by which, in turn, they regulate effector functions of other leukocytes. As in cascade control systems, the network of cell-cell interactions results in a multifaceted cell reaction, whose effectiveness depends on the repertoire of the distinct effector mechanisms turned on. In contrast to the activation of a single effector mechanism, the IL2 based "helper" strategy utilises rIL2 to interfere with the control mechanisms of the immune system [38,38].

We studied the "helper" role of IL2 by transplanting several poorly or non-immunogenic murine tumours into syngeneic mice. A small tumour inhibition was always found when the challenge was followed by 10 daily injections of only 10-20 units (!) of rIL2 around the area of tumour challenge. By contrast, almost complete inhibition took place when these injections were performed in mice challenged with tumour cells admixed with the non-reactive (or suppressed) spleen cells obtained directly from tumour-bearing mice (TB-Ly). This approach, stemming from the association of low doses of IL2 plus non-reactive TB-Ly, was denominated lymphokine-activated tumour inhibition (LATI) [5].

LATI induction starts when relatively low doses of exogenous IL2 bind to receptors of TB-Ly artificially admixed with tumour cells. These receptors are expressed as the result of specific (p75-p55) and nonspecific (p55) recognition of tumour cells. In the presence of exogenous IL2, TB-Ly may acquire LAK activity and kill tumour cells. However, experimental data show that their major role is to secrete and efficiently deliver various lymphokines. In this way, TB-Ly recruit several host lymphocyte populations. These can become directly reactive against the tumour, but can also further amplify the anti-tumour reactivity by releasing, in turn, other lymphokines and chemotactic factors by which they boost endogenous NK activity, activate lymphocyte killer cells and macrophages, attract and activate granulocytes, and induce the expansion of specifically reactive cytolytic and helper T lymphocytes [5,39] The ILs sustaining the inflammatory phase apparently build a favourable milieu for tumour cell recognition and induction of a tumour-specific, systemic and persistent immunity. During tumour growth, T lymphocytes potentially able to specifically interact with tumour become inactive or suppressed. The recognition of tumour cells in the presence of appropriate lymphokines during the nonspecific phases of LATI may induce a significant clonal expansion of these T lymphocytes. The host reac

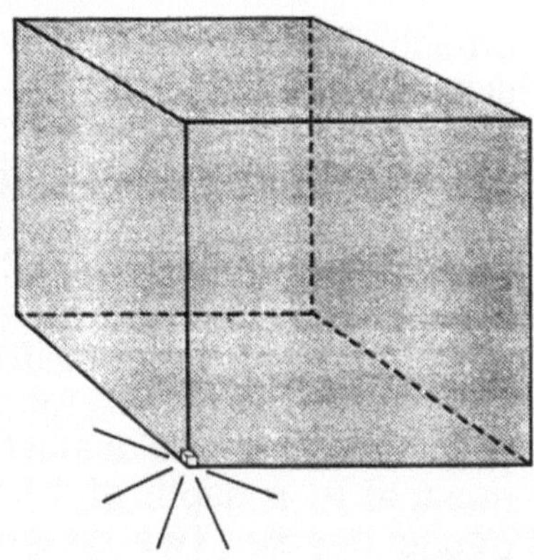

Fig. 3. Comparison between the large doses of IL2 required for an efficient IL2 and LAK (or IL2 only) systemic treatment (large dotted cube), and the locally injected low doses required for LATI-based protocols (small white cube) [26]

tion gradually becomes specific as nonspecific reactivity declines [39].

When LATI is taking place, the tumour growth area is heavily infiltrated by mononuclear cells and granulocytes. Eosinophils are frequent and mostly in close contact with both lymphocytes and tumour cells, suggesting that their cytolytic activity is triggered by factors secreted by activated lymphocytes. Tumour-draining lymph nodes show progressive enlargement with expansion of their cortical and paracortical zones. The wall of epithelioid venules is infiltrated by lymphocytes actively travelling to and from the node. Moreover, mice in which LATI took place 30 days earlier display a tumour-specific delayed-type hypersensitivity, and a significant number of mice acquire a tumour-specific immune memory after LATI [42,39].

The LATI system is a new way of looking at rIL2-mediated immunotherapy, whereby direct reaction to the tumour is elicited by piloting a self-enhancing lymphokine cascade. It may have potential applications in clinical practice, since low doses of IL2 locally injected avoid most of the side-effects associated with systemic injection of large doses (Fig. 3). The experimental results promoted the initiation of clinical trials in recurrent head and neck squamous cell carcinomas, where a treatment based on local stimulation of the immune reactivity of a tumour's satellite lymph nodes appears to be a simple approach. Tumour-draining lymph nodes may substitute TB-Ly.

In an initial trial, 20 patients with recurrent inoperable head and neck squamous cell carcinoma received a course of 10 daily injections of 200 U of natural IL2 (produced by the Jurkat cell line growing in serum-free medium) in 0.5 ml of saline containing 10% human serum albumin, 1.5 cm from the insertion of the sternocleidomastoid muscle on the mastoid to a depth of 1.5 cm, using a 26-gauge needle. Two channels meet at this point and lymphographic studies have shown that injection of radioopaque substances gives excellent visualisation of the local lymphatic network. A response was considered to be complete (CR) if no tumour was evident on direct or optical fibre inspection, partial (PR) if the sum of the products of the longest perpendicular diameters of all lesions decreased by over 50%, and minor (MR) if they decreased by less than 50%.

After a single course, 3 CR (15%), 3 PR (15%) and 8 MR (40%) responses were observed. These subjects presented lymph node enlargement, necrotic sputum and a decrease in the tumour mass. An interesting observation is that even the presence of contralateral neck lymph nodes only was sufficient to permit tumour shrinkage. A direct toxic effect of IL2 on tumour cells can be ruled out, since no clinical effects were observed in patients who had undergone bilateral lymph node dissection, and since the injections were always performed in the vicinity of the mastoid at the junction of 2 lymphatic channels and not intratumourally. However, these biological findings require a few important clinical qualifications:

- Both CR and PR were temporary. Apparently, the new recurring tumours are less sensitive to further IL2 courses. These impressive tumour regressions thus have no significance for survival.
- Regressions are found with small recurrent tumours only [40,41]. When the same IL2 protocol was applied by the P.H.M. De Mulder group to very large, not-pretreated tumours, no shrinkage was found [43].
- Corroboration of the percentages recorded in this small pilot study is now being sought from multicentric trials.

In another group of trials, IL2 was injected in a similar way before surgery to characterise the cellular component of the immune reaction at the tumour growth site, and to see whether surgery itself is accompanied by complications and toxicity. Histological examination of several tumour fragments and tumour-invaded lymph nodes showed that a marked, uniform reaction pattern was elicited. Neoplastic cells were surrounded by leukocytes in the great majority of fragments. This massive infiltration was often associated with degenerated tumour cells or even necrosis. The infiltrating cells were both lymphocytes and cells with the morphology of NK cells. Massive infiltration of eosinophils was also evident and dominated several fields. Lymph nodes displayed hyperplasia of both cortical and paracortical areas, and epithelioid venules with a thick endothelium infiltrated by lymphocytes and granulocytes. In a few cases, a decrease or disappearance of neoplastic lesions was also documented clinically and histologically [42,43].

Conclusions

The LATI method shows that even extremely low doses of "helper" IL2 may be effective. It is not surprising that these initial clinical results were not universal and only temporary, as the advanced head and neck tumours treated were not likely to respond. At present, the use of IL2 in the elicitation of cytotoxic lymphocytes to be passively transferred into tumour-bearing organisms provides important clinical results.

Despite the apparent theoretical simplicity of this approach, the real mechanisms causing tumour shrinkage are still unclear. Quite apart from the comparative effectiveness of killer and helper strategies, our suspicion is that in most cases helper manoeuvres alone are rational, if not the only ones able to have a significant effect on *in vivo* manipulation of the immune reactivity to neoplasia (37,38). IL2-activated cytotoxic T lymphocytes, and LAK cells plus IL2, may induce tumour regression not because of their straight killing power, but rather because of their regulatory activity due to localised delivery of lymphokines, by which they ultimately trigger tumour-specific immunity and pilot a typical lymphokine and cell-mediated cascade-like reaction.

Acknowledgements

We thank Dr. J. Iliffe for careful review of the manuscript. The experimental work of our laboratory reviewed in this paper was supported by grants from the Italian Association for Cancer Research (AIRC), and ISS Italy-USA project for tumour therapy.

REFERENCES

1   Mitchison NA: Regulation of the immune response to cell surface antigens. In: Pernis and Vogel (eds): Regulatory T lymphocytes. Academic Press, New York 1980 pp 147-157

2   Jerne NK, Roland J, Cazenave PA: Recurrent idiotopes and internal images. EMBO J 1982 (1):243-248

3   Janeway CA, Bottomly K, Horowitz J, Kaye J, Jones B, and Tite J: Modes of cell:cell communication in the immune system. J Immunol 1985 (135):739-742

4   Smith KA: Interleukin-2 inception, impact and implications. Science 1988 (240):1169-1174

5   Forni G, Giovarelli M, Santoni A, Modesti A and Forni M: Tumour inhibition by interleukin-2 at the tumour-host interface. Biochim Biophy Acta 1986 (865):307-327

6   Forni G, Santoni A and Giovarelli M: Lymphokine-activated tumor inhibition in vivo. I. The local administration of Interleukin-2 triggers non reactive lymphocytes from tumor bearing mice to inhibit tumor growth. J Immunol 1985 (134):1305-1311

7   Phillips JH, Takeshita T, Sugamura K and Lanier LL: Activation of Natural Killer cells via the p75 interleukin 2 receptor. J Exp Med 1989 (170):291-296

8   Waldmann TA: Multichain Interleukin-2 receptor: A target for immunotherapy in lymphoma. JNCI 1989 (81):914-923

9   Forni G and Giovarelli M: Tumor immunotherapy with interleukin 2 and leukocytes. In: den Otter W, Ruitenberg EJ (eds): Tumor Immunology: Mechanisms, Diagnosis, Therapy. Elsevier Science Publishers, Amsterdam 1987 pp 266-282

10 Kuffer A, Swain SL, Janeway CJ and Singer SJ: The specific direct interactions of helper T and antigen-presenting B cells. Proc Natl Acad Sci USA 1987 (83):6080-6084

11 Forni G: LAK-cells in cancer therapy. A critical assessment, E.O.S. (In press 1989)

12 Cerottini JC and Brunner KT: Cell-mediated cytotoxicity, allograft rejection, and tumor immunity. Adv Immunol 1984 (18):67-79

13 Engers HD, Glasebrook AL and Sorenson GD: Allogeneic tumor rejection induced by the intravenous injection of Lyt.2$^+$ cytolytic T lymphocyte clones. J Exp Med 1982 (156):1280-1286

14 Cheever M, Greenberg PD, Fefer A and Gillis S: Augmentation of the antitumor therapeutic efficacy of long-term cultured T lymphocytes by in vivo administration of purified interleukin-2. J Exp Med 1982 (155):968-978

15 Celada F: Quantitative studies of the adoptive immunological memory in mice. I. An age dependent barrier to syngeneic transplantation. J Exp Med 1966 (124):1-14

16 North RJ: The murine antitumor response and its therapeutic manipulation. Adv Immunol 1984 (35):89-156

17 Hewitt HB: Animal tumor models for tumor immunology. J Biol Resp Modif 1982 (1):107-119

18 Nossal GJV: The case history of Mr. T.I. - Terminal patient or still curable ? - Immunol Today 1980 (1):5-6

19 Herberman RB: Multiple functions of natural killer cells, including immunoregulation as well as resistance to tumor growth. Concepts Immunopathol 1985 (1):96-118

20 Grimm EA and Rosenberg SA: The human lymphokine-activated killer cell phenomenon. The lymphokines 1983 (9):435-442

21 Phillips JH and Lanier LL: Dissection of the lymphokine-activated killer phenomenon. Relative contribution of pheripheral blood natural killer cells and T lymphocytes to cytolysis. J Exp Med 2986 (164):814-825

22 Ortaldo JR : Analysis of lymphokine-activated killer (LAK) cells. In: Truitt RL, Gale RP, Bordin MM (Eds) Cellular Immunotherapy of Cancer. Alan R Liss Inc, New York 1987 p 197

23 Mulé JJ, Shu S, Schwarz SL and Rosenberg SA: Adoptive immunotherapy of established pulmonary metastases with LAK cells and recombinant interleukin-2. Science 1984 (225):1487-1490

24 Lafraniere R and Rosenberg SA: Adoptive immunotherapy of murine hepatic metastases with lymphokine activated killer (LAK) cells and recombinant IL2 can mediate the regression of both immunogenic and non-immunogenic sarcomas and adenocarcinomas . J Immunol 1985 (135):3899-3902

25 Rosenberg SA, Packard BS, Aebersold PM, Solomon P, Topalian SL, Toy ST, Simon P, Lotze MT, Yang JC, Seipp AA, Simpson C, Carter C, Bock S, Schwartzetruber D, Wei JP and White DE: Use of tumor- infiltrating lymphocytes and interleukin-2 in the immunotherapy of patients with metastatic melanoma. N Engl J Med 1988 (319):1676-1680

26 Forni G, Jemma C, Musso T and Giovarelli M: Interleukin-2 in tumor immunology: Biological problems and therapeutic strategies. In: Dammacco F (ed) Recent Adavances in Autoimmunity and Tumor Immunology. Edi-Ermes, Milano 1988 pp 179-198

27 Ettinghausen SE, Puri RK and Rosenberg S: Increased vascular permeability in organ mediated by the systemic administration of lymphokine-activated killer cells and recombinant interleukin-2 in mice. JNCI 1988 (80):177-188

28 Mier JW, Brandon EP, Libby P, Janika MW, and Asonson FR: Activated endothelial cells resist lymphokine-activated killer cell-mediated injury. Possible role of induced cytokines in limiting capillary leak during IL2 therapy. J Immunol 1989 (143):2407-2414

29 Ettinghausen SE, Lipford III EH, Mulé JJ and Rosenberg SA: Systemic administration of recombinant Interleukin-2 stimulated in vivo cell proliferation in tissues. J Immunol 1985 (135):1488-1492

30 Mule JJ, Yang JC and Lafreniere R: Identification of cellular mechanisms operational in vivo during the regression of established pulmonary metatstases by systemic administration of high dose recombinant interleukin-2. J Immunol 1987 (139):285-291

31 Rosenberg SA, Spiess P and Lafreniere R: A new approach to the adoptive immunotherapy of cancer with tumor-infiltrating lymphocytes. Science 1986 (223):1318-1321

32 Rosenberg SA, Packard BS, Aebersold PM, Solomon D, Topalian SL, Toy ST, Simon P, Lotze MT, Yang JC, Seipp CA, Simpson C, Carter C, Bock S, Schwartzentruber D, Wei JP and White DE: Use of tumor-infiltrating lymphocytes and Interleukin-2 in the immunotherapy of patients with metastatic melanoma. N Engl J Med 1988 (319):1676-1680

33 Herberman RB: Animal tumor models and their relevance to human tumor immunology. J Biol Resp Modif 1983 (2):39-46

34 Forni G and Santoni A: Immunogenicity of non-immunogenic tumors. J Biol Resp Modif 1984 (3):128-131

35 Anichini A, Fossati G and Parmiani G: Heterogeneity of clones from a human metastatic melanoma detected by autologous cytotoxic T lymphocyte clones. J Exp Med 1986 (163):215-220

36 West WH, Tauer KW, Yannelli JR, Marshall GD, Orr DW, Thurman GB and Oldham RK: Constant-infusion recombinant interleukin-2 in adoptive immunotherapy of advanced cancer. N Engl J Med 1987 (316):898-892

37 Forni G and Giovarelli M: Strategies for cell-mediated immunotherapy of cancer: killing or help? Immunology Today 1986 (7):202-203

38 Forni G, Fujiwara H, Martino F, Hamaoka T, Jemma C, Caretto P and Giovarelli M: Helper strategy in tumor immunology: expansion of helper lymphocytes and utilization of helper lymphokines for experimental and clinical immunotherapy. Cancer Metastasis Rev 1988 (7): 289-309

39 Forni G, Musso T, Jemma C, Boraschi D, Tagliabue A, Giovarelli M: Lymphokine activated tumor inhibition (LATI) in mice: ability of a nonapeptide of the human Interleukin-1 to recruit antitumor reactivity in recipient mice. J Immunol 1989 (142):712-718

40 Cortesina G, De Stefani A, Giovarelli M, Barioglio MG, Cavallo GP, Jemma CC and Forni G: Treatment of recurrent squamous cell carcinoma of head and neck with low doses of interleukin-2 (IL2) injected perilymphatically. Cancer 1988 (62): 2482-2485

41 Forni G, Giovarelli M, Jemma C, Bosco MC, Caretto P, Modesti A, Santoni A, Forni M, Cortesina G, De Steafani A, Cavallo GP, Galeazzi E, Musiani P, De Campora E, Valitutti S, Castellino F, Calearo CV, Fontana G, Sesia G: Perilymphatic injections of cytokines: A new tool in active cancer immunotherapy. Experimental rationale and clinical findings. Ann Ist Sup Sanita' (In press 1989)

42 Forni G, Giovarelli M, Jemma C, Bosco MC, Cortesina G, De Stefani A, Cavallo G, Forni M, Boraschi D, Musiani P: Injections of Interleukins around tumor-draining lymph nodes: a new mode of immunotherapy. In Schirrmacher V, Schwartz-Albiez R (eds) Cancer Metastasis. Springer Verlag, Berlin 1989 pp 181-185

43 De Mulder PHM, Schornagel JH, Ruiter DJ, Van den Broek P, Hordijk G, Verweij J, Knegt P, and Galatzka A: A phase II study of perilymphatically injected recombinant interleukin-2 in locally far advanced, non-pretreated head and neck squamous cell carcinoma. Abstract 6th NCI EORTC Symposium on New Drugs in Cancer Therapy. Amsterdam 1989

44 Musiani P, De Campora P, Valitutti S, Castellino F, Calearo CV, Jemma C, De Stefani A, Forni G: Effect of low doses of interleukin-2 injected perilymphatically and peritumorally in patients with advanced primary head and neck squamous cell carcinoma. J Biol Resp Modif 1989 (8):571-578

Cellular Immunotherapy of Cancer: The Use of Lymphokine-Activated Natural Killer (LANAK) Cells

Françoise Farace [1], Bernard Escudier [2], Frédéric Triebel [1] and Thierry Hercend [1]

1 Laboratoire d'Hémato-Immunologie, INSERM U333, Institut Gustave Roussy, rue Camille Desmoulins, Villejuif 94805, France
2 Service de Réanimation, Institut Gustave Roussy, rue Camille Desmoulins, Villejuif 94805, France

"Active immunotherapy" of cancer has been defined as the stimulation of the host immune system aimed at rejection of the tumour. In recent years, this has been the principal subject of research in this field. Attempts have been made to either immunise patients with allogeneic tumour cells, or to increase their immune responses more generally by non-specific stimulation with, for example, BCG or interferons [1]. These early trials were most often disappointing, with a few exceptions, such as the local use of BCG in the early stage of bladder carcinoma [2]. Recently, the development of clinical trials with IL2, which is a pivotal mediator of the immune system, has led to a renewed interest in active immunotherapy. Indeed, infusions of high-dose IL2 have been shown to induce partial and even complete responses in a substantial proportion (20-30%) of patients with metastatic renal cell carcinoma and melanoma [3]. An additional approach is represented by "adoptive immunotherapy", i.e., the transfer of immunologically active agents to the patient. Along these lines, one method has been studied extensively in recent years; it is based on the *in-vivo* infusion of cells displaying *in-vitro* antitumour cytotoxic activity. In 1980, S. Rosenberg and co-workers at the United States National Cancer Institute showed that the treatment of murine splenocytes with supernatants containing IL2 resulted in the generation of cells able to kill a wide variety of fresh tumour targets, but not normal cells [4]. These lymphocytes were termed LAK (Lymphokine Activated Killer) cells. Subsequent studies in various animal models have shown that, under certain conditions, the transfusion of such killer lymphocytes may lead to the regression of established metastases. We shall briefly summarise here the data from these murine experiments, as well as the initial clinical results obtained when the method based on the animal models was tested in humans. We shall then discuss the current problems related to this approach and the potential developments for the future.

Animal Models

Animal studies have played a direct and critical role as the basis for the clinical development of adoptive immunotherapy. The essential findings of this extensive experimentation can be summarised as follows:
- Three days' *in-vitro* IL2 incubation of normal murine splenocytes is optimal for LAK-cell generation (i.e., an optimal cytotoxic activity is detected against a series of genetically unrelated tumour cell lines) [5].
- LAK cells alone infused into tumour-bearing animals do not induce tumour regression [6,7].
- IL2 alone is also generally inefficacious. However, in some models, including sarcoma and melanoma, IL2 infusions displayed a degree of antitumour activity

when performed at very high, toxic doses. In this case, the generation of LAK cells was detected in the spleen of the recipient mice [8].

- Regression of established pulmonary and hepatic metastases can be commonly obtained using a combined treatment with both IL2 infusions and LAK-cell transfusions [6,9,10].
- LAK-cell plus IL2 therapy induces regression of tumours of distinct histological types such as sarcomas, melanomas and colon adenocarcinomas [6,7,10,11].
- The effect of therapy is dependent upon the dose of both LAK cells and IL2 [7].
- Allogeneic LAK cells are almost as effective as syngeneic LAK cells [7].
- The LAK-cell/IL2 treatment remains efficacious when one destroys the immune system of the recipient animal by various methods including chemotherapy, irradiation or more complex procedures such as the generation of so-called B mice (thymectomised, irradiated and subsequently reconstituted with T-cell depleted bone marrow) [7,8,12].
- Adoptively transferred LAK cells divide *in vivo* when IL2 is administered concomitantly [13]. Irradiated LAK cells are ineffective [7], suggesting that an intact proliferation potential in the presence of IL2 is required for the expression of the therapeutic effect.

In conclusion, it was found that the addition of *in-vitro* IL2-activated lymphocytes to the lymphokine infusions was generally required to increase the response rates and to improve the quality of tumour regression. The finding that IL2/LAK-cell treatment induces antitumour responses in immunodepleted animals strongly suggested that the beneficial effects are, for the most part, adoptive. The overall rationale deriving from these studies is that the transfused cells are the critical effectors of the antitumour response, this activity being, however, dependent upon their activation maintained *in vivo* by the IL2 infusions.

One way to increase the efficacy of cellular immunotherapy is to infuse suspensions with potentially improved antitumour activity on a per-cell basis. *In vitro*, it has been clearly shown that only a small fraction of the so-called LAK cells actually displays a cytotoxic activity against tumour cells. A method to en-

rich LAK cells in cytotoxic effectors has been investigated recently by J.C. Hiserodt and co-workers [14,15]. They have found in both rats and mice that adherent lymphocytes present in the LAK-cell preparations display the highest cytotoxic potential. These adherent LAK cells are usually referred to as "A-LAK" (i.e., Adherent LAK cells). Characterisation of the A-LAK cells has indicated that they are IL2-activated, large, granular lymphocytes (LGL) and thus belong essentially to the NK cell type. It has recently been shown in rats with established pulmonary and hepatic metastases that the administration of A-LAK cells and IL2 is superior to a standard LAK-cell/IL2 treatment with regard to tumour regression and increased survival [16]. Initial studies have been undertaken to characterise human A-LAK cells (see the relevant chapter by R. Herberman).

Another form of adoptive immunotherapy with immune cells is based on the use of lymphocytes which are directly extracted from tumour sites (designated Tumour Infiltrating Lymphocytes or "TIL") and subsequently expanded *in vitro* with IL2. It has been shown that certain TIL suspensions contain tumour-specific α/β^+ MHC-restricted cytotoxic T lymphocytes [17,18]. In several murine tumour models, TIL/IL2 infusions were found to be 100 to 500 times more efficient than their LAK/IL2 counterparts [19]. In these experiments, the antitumour activity of the TIL/IL2-treated mice was potentiated by prior administration of cyclophosphamide.

Clinical Trials

When recombinant IL2 became available, clinical trials were initiated in patients with advanced cancer. As animal models predicted that the administration of LAK cells in conjunction with IL2 would potentially be more efficient than the use of IL2 alone, Rosenberg and co-workers designed a protocol to generate human LAK cells in order to evaluate their clinical usefulness.

The basic protocol that resulted from these studies is the following: patients receive IL2 administration by intravenous bolus every 8 hours for 5 days, followed by a 3-day rest pe-

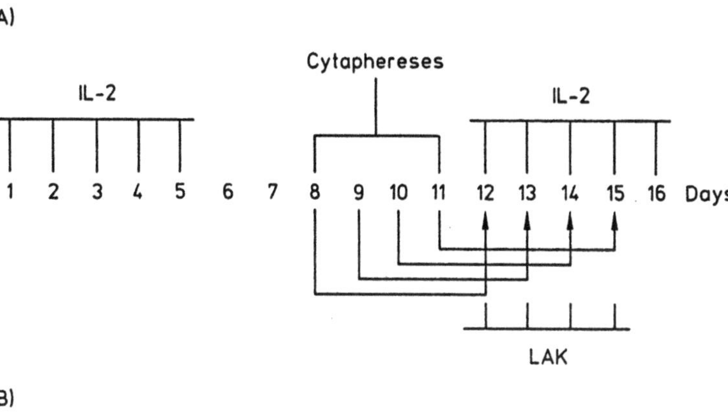

Fig. 1.
Panel 1A. Treatment protocol using rIL2 and LAK cells. Cytapheresis is performed 3 days after the interruption of rIL2 infusions. Harvested PBLs are cultured for 3 to 4 days in the presence of rIL2 to generate LAK cells

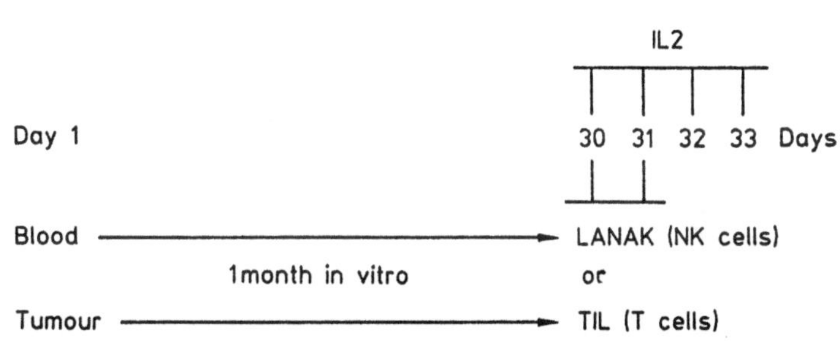

Panel 1B. Treatment protocol using rIL2 and either TIL or LANAK cells. TILs are extracted from the tumour site and amplified for approximately one month before infusion into the patient.
NK cells are purified from patient peripheral blood; they are subsequently activated and amplified approx. 1 month before infusion

riod. The lymphocyte counts decrease during the IL2 infusions and this is followed by a rebound in the lymphocyte numbers 48 hours after the last infusion [20,21]. Taking advantage of this lymphocytosis, 5 daily lymphaphereses are performed and the harvested mononuclear cells are incubated in the presence of IL2 for 3 or 4 days to generate LAK cells. IL2 administration is restarted on the last day with lymphapheresis while LAK-cell infusions are given for an additional 5-day period (Fig. 1A). This treatment is performed either once or twice, depending upon the patients. The preliminary results in a series of 25 patients appeared encouraging [22] and the approach was subsequently tested on a larger scale at the NCI and in many other centres.

The results from the NCI group, which has the widest experience in immunotherapy, have been updated recently [3]. Six hundred and fifty-two patients with resistant metastatic tumours, mostly (73%) malignant melanoma or renal cell carcinoma, received various biological treatments between November 1984 and March 1989. In this series, 130 evaluable patients were treated by rIL2 alone, with a response rate of 22% in renal cell carcinoma and 24% in melanoma. No objective responses were seen in 34 patients with other histological types, when using IL2 alone. One hundred and seventy-seven evaluable patients were treated by rIL2 and LAK cells, with a response rate of 35% in renal cell carcinoma and 21% in melanoma. Five objective responses were seen in 30 patients with metastatic colorectal cancer and 4 in 7 patients with non-Hodgkin's lymphoma. Of 18 patients in complete remission who were treated either with IL2 alone (4 out of 130) or with LAK/IL2 (14 out of 177), 10 have remained disease free with a follow-up of 10 to 52 months.

In previous, non-randomised trials, there was no clear correlation between the number of transfused LAK cells, their lytic potential and clinical outcome [23-25]. Thus, the recent study by Rosenberg et al. (quoted in ref. 3), which is at present the only known randomised trial comparing the efficacy of IL2 alone versus IL2 plus LAK cells, shows a borderline advantage in favour of the cellular treatment. Indeed, although the overall response rates are similar in the two regimens, the incidence of complete responses is greater in patients who received LAK cells plus IL2.

Infusions of IL2-activated TIL cells have also been performed in humans, mainly in melanoma patients. The infiltrating lymphocytes are isolated from enzymatic digests and expanded *in vitro* in the presence of IL2 for approximately 4 weeks (Fig. 1B). In most cases, the patients received these TIL suspensions as a single infusion while IL2 administration was started immediately after cell administration and continued at high doses for several days. In preliminary studies, 11 of the 20 treated patients showed objective responses [19]. However, the duration of the responses was generally short and only one of the responders had a complete remission.

Rationale for Immunotherapy with LANAK Cells and rIL2

As briefly summarised here, immunotherapy with IL2-cultured cells and lymphokine infusion has proven effective for the eradication of metastatic tumours in experimental animals. The clinical trials based on these models have confirmed that IL2 is indeed an active agent in a currently limited number of tumour types, including melanoma and renal cell carcinoma. However, the contribution of cell infusions to tumour regression when used in addition to IL2 has appeared less substantial than could have been expected from pre-clinical experimentation. In fact, analysis of the clinical literature [3,23-25] supports the view that the adoptive effects due to cell infusions are much less dramatic in humans, even though they may increase the efficacy of the treatment. Thus, the future of this approach is questionable since it is highly demanding with respect to both labour and cost. To be pursued as a practical therapeutic modality, it should be improved in order to generate substantially better clinical results. As pointed out, this would require the testing of cell suspensions potentially more efficacious than the LAK cultures.

Using TIL preparations is one possible solution. However, there are a number of limitations hampering this development. The first and most evident is that sufficiently large tumour samples (in practice from superficial metastases) have to be available. Indeed, it appears likely from the murine data that efficacy is dependent upon the number of cells that can be produced and infused following

in-vitro expansion from the tumour fragments [19]. Perhaps more importantly, it is not yet clear whether the rationale underlying the use of TIL will be relevant for human tumours. The major point of this rationale is that TIL cultures from murine models contain conventional MHC-restricted tumour-specific CTL. Thus far, analogous human T lymphocytes have been identified by cell cloning in certain melanomas exclusively [17,26,27]. The unequivocal demonstration that such effectors are present in other human tumour types is still awaited. Moreover, the large-scale TIL melanoma cultured cells which were actually infused into patients were found in most cases to display MHC-unrestricted cytolytic activity (as opposed to MHC-restricted CTL activity) [28]. These data support the view that, even though conventional CTLs may be present in the tumour and subsequently in the "TIL suspensions", their frequency is probably very low. Finally, it is doubtful that the exclusive use of specific CTLs would be curative. Indeed, it is known that tumours are heterogeneous and contain mutants that are likely to escape the specific responses directed at unique peptidic fragments of tumour-associated antigens. Together, it is certainly of interest to pursue studies on TIL infusions in order better to characterise these lymphocytes and assess their *in-vivo* activity, with particular respect to biodistribution and homing. Reinfused specific CTLs may indeed concentrate better at the tumour sites than non-specific effectors [29]. However, it is unlikely that this strategy will generalise until lymphocyte responses engaged locally at the tumour site are better understood.

Improvement of suspensions used in cellular immunotherapy can also be attempted through the development of cultures enriched in effectors with broad antitumour activity present in peripheral blood. *In-vitro* studies performed in humans have shown that the antitumour activity of LAK preparations is mediated in a virtually exclusive fashion by a small fraction of CD3- CD56+ (NKH1+) CD16+ Natural Killer (NK) cells [30,31]. These IL2-activated NK effectors generally represent less than 10% of the cells present in the LAK cultures, while most of the remaining T lymphocytes have no antitumour activity detectable *in vitro*. It should be noted, however, that minor fractions of CD3+ T lymphocytes present in IL2-activated peripheral blood mononuclear cells (PBMC) can display non-MHC requiring cytotoxic activity against tumour cells, but this contribution is usually very limited [32-34]. To improve the efficacy of blood-derived cell infusions, our approach has thus been to design experimental conditions appropriate for the generation of highly purified preparations of Lymphokine Activated Natural Killer (LANAK) cells.

In preliminary experiments, we investigated different procedures of purification. Attempts to purify positively peripheral NK cells were hampered by the relatively weak expression of the NKH1 and CD16 molecules. We therefore tested a negative selection approach using procedures based on either panning, immuno-rosetting or complement-dependent cytotoxicity. Immuno-rosetting appeared to be the most efficient and reproducible method. Briefly, non-adherent mononuclear cells are treated with a mixture of monoclonal antibodies directed at B lymphocytes (anti-CD19, anti-MHC class II), T lymphocytes (anti-CD3, anti-CD4, anti-CD8, anti-TCR α/β, anti-TCR γ/δ) and monocytes (anti-CD14, anti-MHC class II). Immunomagnetic beads are used to form rosettes with the positive cells, and the non-rosetted fraction containing the NK lymphocytes is recovered. Two successive cycles of purification using the mixture of monoclonal antibodies are performed. The purity of the non-rosetting fraction is controlled morphologically, LGL being found to represent 85% to 90% of the purified cells. These lymphocytes are then cultured in V bottom microtiter plates. The feeder layer is made of irradiated lymphoblastoid cells and allogeneic PBMC. Cultures are fed with recombinant IL2 and crude leucocyte-conditioned medium (LCM). Phenotypic analysis of the expanding lymphocytes is performed with a series of monoclonal antibodies. These procedures lead to the development of highly purified LANAK cells with less than 5% CD3+ contaminating T lymphocytes and a reactivity with anti-NKH1 greater than 95%. Multiple alterations of the culture method described here, which has been used for many years to generate and maintain human NK clones, have been attempted unsuccessfully. Thus, the conventional culture method [35] has simply been scaled up to generate large cell numbers appropriate for clinical infusions.

Feasibility Trial with LANAK Cells and rIL2 in Metastatic Renal Cell Carcinoma

Metastatic renal cell carcinoma was selected as a relevant clinical situation for testing LANAK cells because initial reports suggested that the administration of LAK suspensions in association with IL2 could improve the clinical responses [36]. As mentioned, the recent randomised trial conducted by Rosenberg et al. further supported this view [3].

The feasibility of generating large numbers of LANAK cells has been tested as follows: one peripheral blood sample (50 to 150 ml) is drawn from each patient on day 1, and CD3⁻ NK lymphocytes are purified by immuno-rosetting (Fig. 2). Approximately 1 to 2×10^6 cells are usually obtained in the non-rosetted fraction and cultured on 1 or 2 microplates. The generation of 20×10^6 cells requires a mean of 8 days. At this step, cells are harvested and an additional round of purification by immuno-rosetting is performed. The negative fraction is expanded on 20 microplates and cultured for 6 to 8 days until approximately 400×10^6 LANAK cells are generated (day 14 in Fig. 2). A fraction of these lymphocytes is used directly for large-scale expansion while the remaining cells are frozen to be used for a second course of treatment. For each cycle of cellular therapy, 200×10^6 LANAK cells are further cultured on 300 microplates for an additional 9 to 12 days. These large-scale amplifications are performed with an automatic device (Biomek 1000, Beckman) driven by an IBM computer with various appropriate programmes. Cells harvested from microplates are transferred in 5 to 20 culture bags, checked by a series of bacteriological controls, and cultured for an additional period of 2 to 5 days prior to infusion.

In most cases, highly pure LANAK cell suspensions of relevant NK cell phenotype were

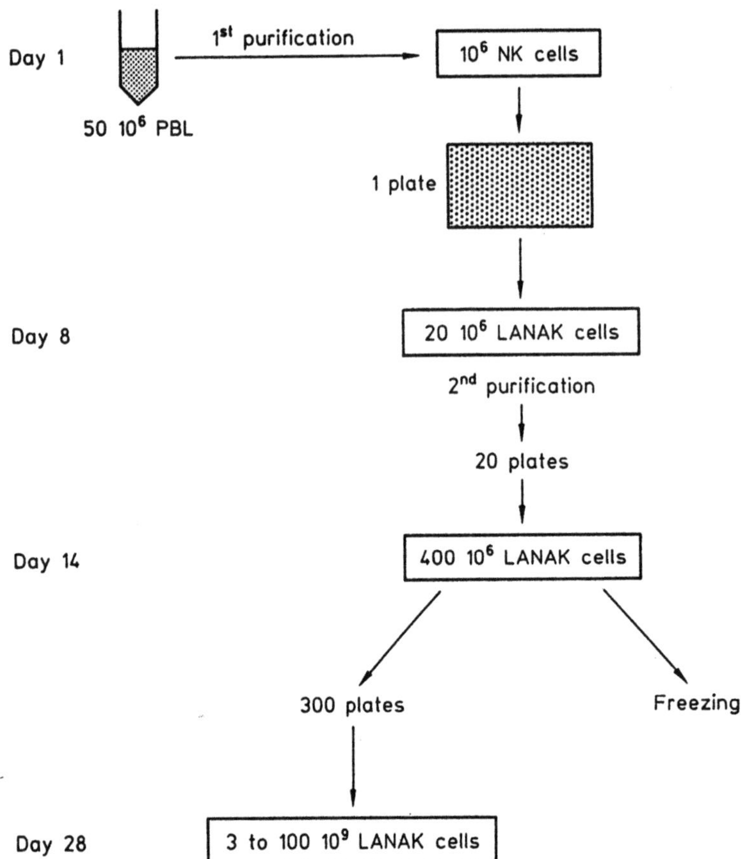

Fig. 2. Amplification protocol of LANAK cells. NK cells are purified on day 1 from peripheral blood and on day 8 from the initial *in vitro* cultures. LANAK cells are subsequently amplified on multiple microplates with irradiated feeder layer and IL2. They are infused into the patient following a 4 to 5-week culture period

obtained. This point is exemplified in Table 1 which displays the phenotype of LANAK cell suspensions that were infused into 5 patients. As shown, cells were CD2+, CD3-, TCR α/β-, TCR γ/δ-, CD4-, partially CD8+ (dull) and NKH1+. The *in-vitro* cytotoxic potential of LANAK cells has been compared to that of autologous LAK cells. For this purpose, PBMCs of the IL2-treated patients were isolated at the peak of lymphocytosis as in standard LAK protocols and then frozen. In parallel, samples of LANAK cells were frozen prior

Table 1. Immunofluorescence analysis of infused LANAK cells

	% positive cells				
MoAb	Patient 1	Patient 2	Patient 3	Patient 4	Patient 5
NKH1*	86	59	85	64	94
CD2	93	93	83	93	96
CD3	1	1	1	12	2
CD4	1	2	3	1	1
CD8	2	1	5	2	7
BMA031	1	1	1	3	11
TcRδ1	1	3	1	13	5

Shown are the % of positive cells for the indicated markers
* The fluorescence intensity obtained with anti-NKH1 was weak in certain cultures, without clearcut distinctions between the positive and negative cell fractions

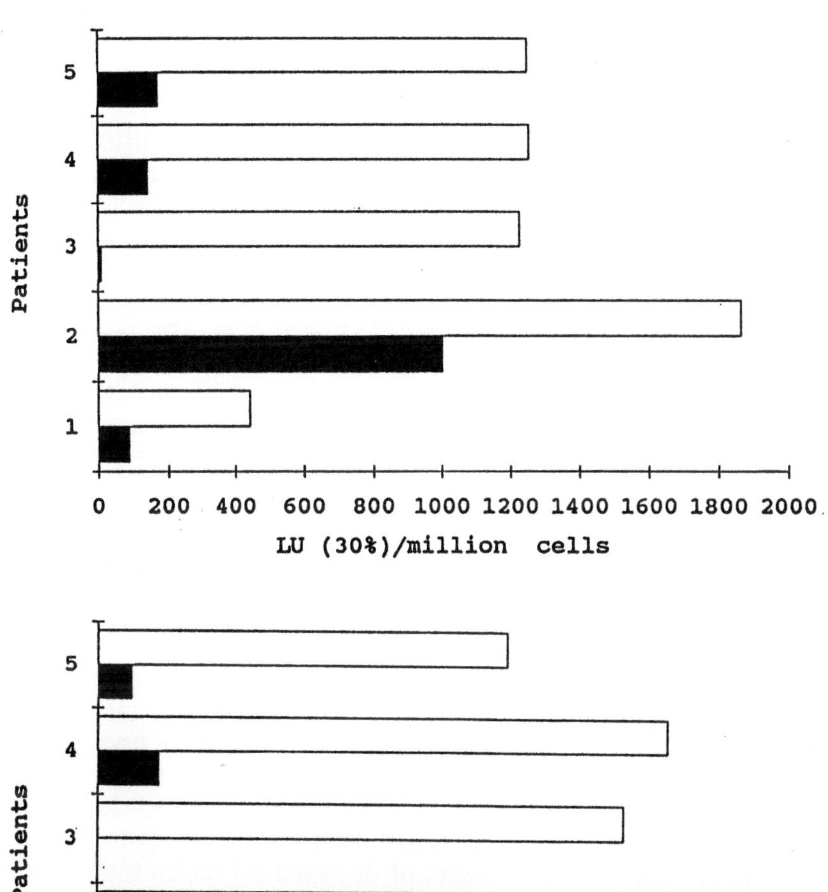

Fig. 3. Comparative cytotoxic activity of LAK (shaded bars) and LANAK (open bars) against K562 (top panel) and DAUDI targets (bottom panel) of 5 patients

to infusion. For each patient, both LAK and LANAK fractions were thawed, cultured in IL2 for 3 days under identical conditions and tested in the same experiment against K562 and DAUDI cells. As an example, the cytotoxicity of LAK and LANAK cells of 5 patients is presented in Figure 3. The *in-vitro* cytotoxic potential of LANAK cells was always greater than that of their LAK counterparts. As shown, LANAK cells were 2 to 100 times and 2 to 1,000 times more effective than LAK cells against K562 lysis and DAUDI, respectively. In addition, there was less variability of the cy-

totoxic potential from one patient to another in the LANAK-cell suspensions.

Twelve patients with a histologically proven diagnosis of metastatic renal cell cancer were included in the study. Given the presence of irradiated lymphoblastoid cells in the feeder layers, only patients with serum IgG antibodies directed to the viral capside antigen (VCA) of Epstein Barr virus (EBV) were eligible. According to the Eurocetus renal cell carcinoma protocol, 2 courses of treatment were scheduled at 3-weekly intervals. Each course included 2 periods of rIL2 (5 days and 4 days) administered by 24-hour continuous infusion

$(3 \times 10^6 U/m^2/d)$ and LANAK cells were infused during the second period. The number of cells infused ranged from 7 to 125×10^9. Nine patients treated with 2 courses of rIL2 and LANAK cells were evaluable. Partial remission was observed in 3 patients. Regarding toxicity, the only feature noted was infrequent episodes of chills. In addition, no increase in serum anti-EBV antigen-related titers was observed.

Some relevant information has been obtained from this study. Only a few patients were treated and one cannot draw any conclusions regarding the efficacy, although the development of 3 PR out of 9 evaluable patients is encouraging. Large amounts of LANAK cells were infused without any apparent toxicity, supporting the view that IL2-activated NK lymphocytes have little, if any, lytic activity against normal tissues *in vivo*. In these immunodepressed, often lymphopenic, patients, quantitative LANAK cell production has been heterogeneous. Moreover, the procedures used to generate pure LANAK lymphocytes are labour- and material-intensive and relatively complex. In an attempt to reduce the length of the culture and to obtain better reproducibility in the LANAK cell production, we are currently purifying larger numbers of NK cells (10^8 instead of 10^6) prior to the cultures. For this purpose, 1 round of cytapheresis is now introduced on day 1 and it is expected that equivalent numbers of LANAK cells can be generated in 12/14 days, thus substantially reducing cost and effort. Increased automation of the cultures will also help to achieve this goal.

Conclusions

Novel forms of cancer immunotherapy are now developing into a multifaceted area of clinical research, including the improvement of IL2 infusion schedules, the association of IL2 with other lymphokines and the combination of these biological therapies with conventional cancer treatments. The relevance of cellular therapy in this context remains questionable because initial clinical results have suggested that adoptive effects are less pronounced in clinical situations than in experimental models. However, virtually all the trials were performed with highly heterogeneous cell fractions and the actual lymphocyte subsets (specific CTL, LANAK, A-LAK, which are now being tested in humans) which will provide the best contribution to tumour regression in given clinical situations are not yet defined. Ideally, one would hope that cytokine-based therapy combined with conventional treatments may suppress the need for cellular transfers which are complex and demanding. Yet, it is reasonable to believe that improving the treatment of resistant metastatic cancers will still require, for a long time, the combined use of every possible means potentially able to induce tumour regression. Thus, refinements of cellular immunotherapy methods should be carefully tested.

Acknowledgement

This work was supported in part by the ADRC grant No 6338 and the IGR grant CRC 8D12.

REFERENCES

1 Oliver RTD: The clinical potential of interleukin-2. Br J Cancer 1988 (58):405-409

2 Pinsky CM, Camacho FJ, Kerr D, Geller NL, Klein FA, Herr HA, Whitmore WF and Oettgen HF: Intravesical administration of Bacillus Calmette-Guerin in patients with recurrent superficial carcinoma of the urinary bladder: report of a prospective, randomized trial. Cancer Treat Rep 1985 (69):47-53

3 Rosenberg SA, Lotze MT, Yang JC, Aebersold PM, Linehan WM, Seipp C and White DE: Experience with the use of high-dose Interleukin-2 in the treatment of 652 cancer patients. Ann Surg 1989 (210):474-485

4 Lotze MT, Grimm EA, Mazumder A, Strausser JL and Rosenberg SA: Lysis of fresh and cultured autologous tumor by human lymphocytes cultured in T-cell growth factor. Cancer Res 1981 (41):4420-4425

5 Rosenberg S: Lymphokine-activated killer cells: A new approach to immunotherapy of cancer. JNCI 1985 (75):595-603

6 Mulé JJ, Shu S, Schwarz SL and Rosenberg SA: Adoptive immunotherapy of established pulmonary metastases with LAK cells and recombinant Interleukin-2. Science 1984 (225):1487-1489

7 Mulé JJ, Shu S and Rosenberg SA: The anti-tumor efficacy of lymphokine-activated killer cells and recombinant interleukin 2 in vivo. J Immunol 1985 (135):646-652

8 Rosenberg SA, Mulé JJ, Spiess PJ, Reichert CM and Schwarz SL: Regression of established pulmonary metastases and subcutaneous tumor mediated by the systemic administration of high-dose recombinant interleukin 2. J Exp Med 1985 (161):1169-1188

9 Lafreniere R and Rosenberg SA: Successful immunotherapy of murine experimental hepatic metastases with lymphokine-activated killer cells and recombinant interleukin 2. Cancer Res 1985 (45):3735-3741

10 Lafreniere R and Rosenberg SA: Adoptive immunotherapy of murine hepatic metastases with lymphokine activated killer (LAK) cells and recombinant Interleukin 2 (RIL 2) can mediate the regression of both immunogenic and nonimmunogenic sarcomas and an adenocarcinoma. J Immunol 1985 (135):4273-4280

11 Papa MZ, Mule JJ and Rosenberg SA: Antitumor efficacy of lymphokine-activated killer cells and recombinant interleukin 2 in vivo: successful immunotherapy of established pulmonary metastases from weakly immunogenic and nonimmunogenic murine tumors of three distinct histological types. Cancer Res 1986 (46):4973-4978

12 Mulé JJ, Yang J, Shu S and Rosenberg SA: The anti-tumor efficacy of lymphokine-activated killer cells and recombinant Interleukin 2 in vivo: direct correlation between reduction of established metastases and cytolytic activity of lymphokine-activated killer cells. J Immunol 1986 (136):3899-3909

13 Ettinghausen SE, Lipford EH, Mule JJ and Rosenberg SA: Systemic administration of recombinant interleukin 2 stimulates in vivo lymphoid cell proliferation in tissues. J Immunol 1985 (135):1488-1497

14 Al Maghazachi A, Vujanovic NL, Herberman RB and Hiserodt JC: Lymphokine-activated killer cells in rats. IV. Developmental relationships among large agranular lymphocytes, large granular lymphocytes, and lymphokine-activated killer cells. J Immunol 1988 (140):2846-2852

15 Vujanovic NL, Herberman RB, Al Maghazachi A and Hiserodt JC: Lymphokine-activated killer cells in rats. III. A simple method for the purification of large granular lymphocytes and their rapid expansion and conversion into lymphokine-activated killer cells . J Exp Med 1988 (167):15-29

16 Schwarz RE, Vujanovic NL and Hiserodt JC: Enhanced antimetastatic activity of lymphokine-activated killer cells purified and expaned by their adherence to plastic. Cancer Res 1989 (49):1441-1446

17 Itoh K, Platsoucas CD and Balch CM: Autologous tumor-specific cytotoxic T lymphocytes in the infiltrate of human metastatic melanomas: Activation by Interleukin 2 and autologous tumor cells, and involvement of the T cell receptor. J Exp Med 1988 (168):1419-1441

18 Topalian SL, Solomon D and Rosenberg SA: Tumor-specific cytolysis by lymphocytes infiltrating human melanomas. J Immunol 1989 (142):3714-3725

19 Rosenberg SA, Spiess P and Lafreniere R: A new approach to the adoptive immunotherapy of cancer with tumor-infiltrating lymphocytes. Science 1986 (233):1318-1321

20 Lotze MT, Matory YL, Ettinghausen SE, Rayner AA, Sharrow SO, Seipp CAY, Custer MC and Rosenberg SA: In vivo administration of purified human interleukin 2. II. Half-life, immunologic effects, and expansion of peripheral lymphoid cells in vivo with recombinant IL2. J Immunol 1985 (135):2865-2875

21 Lotze MT, Frana LW, Sharrow SO, Robb RJ and Rosenberg SA: In vivo administration of purified human interleukin 2. I. Half-life and immunologic effects of the Jurkat cell line-derived interleukin 2. J Immunol 1985 (134):157-166

22 Rosenberg SA, Lotze MT, Muul LM, Leitman S, Chang AE, Ettinghausen SE, Matory YL, Skibber JM, Shiloni E, Vetto JT, Seipp CA, Simpson C and Reichert CM: Observations of the systemic administration of autologous lymphokine-activated killer cells and recombinant Interleukin-2 to patients with metastatic cancer. N Engl J Med 1985 (313):1485-1492

23 West WH, Tauer KW, Yannelli JR, Marshall GD, Orr DW, Thurman GB and Oldham RK: Constant-infusion recombinant Interleukin-2 in adoptive immunotherapy of advanced cancer. N Engl J Med 1987 (136):898-905

24 Dutcher JP, Creekmore S, Weiss GR, Margolin K, Markowitz AB, Roper M, Parkinson D, Ciobanu N, Fisher RI, Boldt DH, Doroshow JH, Rayner AA, Hawkins M and Atkins M: A phase II study of interleukin-2 and lymphokine-activated killer cells in

patients with metastatic malignant melanoma. J Clin Oncol 1989 (7):477-485

25 Fisher RI, Coltman CA, Doroshow JH, Rayner AA, Hawkins MJ, Mier JW, Wiernik P, McMannis JD, Weiss GR, Margolin KA, Gemlo BT, Hoth DF, Parkinson DR and Paietta E: Metastatic renal cancer treated with interleukin-2 and lymphokine-activated killer cells. Ann Intern Med 1988 (108):518-523

26 Anichini A, Mazzocchi A, Fossati G and Parmiani G: Cytotoxic T lymphocyte clones from peripheral blood and from tumor site detect intratumor heterogeneity of melanoma cells. Analysis of specificity and mechanisms of interaction. J Immunol 1989 (142):3692-3701

27 Mukherji B, Guha A, Chakraborty NG, Sivanandham M, Nashed AL, Sporn JR and Ergin MT: Clonal analysis of cytotoxic and regulatory T cell responses against human melanoma. J Exp Med 1989 (169):1961-1976

28 Topalian SL, Solomon D, Avis FP, Chang AE, Freerksen DL, Linehan WM, Lotze MT, Robertson CN, Seipp CA, Simon P, Simpson CG and Rosenberg SA: Immunotherapy of patients with advanced cancer using tumor-infiltrating lymphocytes and recombinant Interleukin-2: a pilot study. J Clin Oncol 1988 (6):839-853

29 Fisher B, Packard BS, Read EJ, Carrasquillo JA, Carter CS, Topalian SL, Yang JC, Yolles P, Larson SM and Rosenberg SA: Tumor localization of adoptively transferred indium-111 labeled tumor infiltrating lymphocytes in patients with metastatic melanoma. J Clin Oncol 1989 (7):250-261

30 Ortaldo JR, Mason A and Overton R: Lymphokine-activated killer cells: Analysis of progenitors and effectors . J Exp Med 1986 (164):1193-1205

31 Phillips JH and Lanier LL: Dissection of the lymphokine-activated killer phenomenon: relative contribution of peripheral blood natural killer cells and T lymphocytes to cytolysis. J Exp Med 1986 (164):814-825

32 Hercend T, Reinherz EL, Meuer SC, Schlossman SF and Ritz J: Phenotypic and functional heterogeneity of human cloned natural killer cell lines. Nature 1983 (301):158-160

33 Hercend T and Schmidt RE: Characteristics and uses of natural killer cells. Immunol Today 1988 (9):291-292

34 Patel SS, Thiele DL and Lipsky PE: Major histocompatibility complex-unrestricted cytolytic activity of human T cells. J Immunol 1987 (139):3886-3895

35 Hercend T, Meuer S, Reinherz EL, Schlossman SF and Ritz J: Generation of a cloned NK cell line derived from the null cell fraction of human peripheral blood. J Immunol 1982 (129):1299-1305

36 Rosenberg SA, Lotze MT, Muul LM, Chang AE, Avis FP, Leitman S, Linehan WM, Robertson CN, Lee RE, Rubin JT, Seipp CA, Simpson CG and White DE: A progress report on the treatment of 157 patients with advanced cancer using lymphokine-activated killer cells and Interleukin-2 or high-dose Interleukin-2 alone. N Engl J Med 1987 (316):889-897

Interleukin 2: Clinical Aspects

N. Thatcher

Cancer Research Campaign, Department of Medical Oncology, Christie Hospital and Holt Radium Institute, Manchester M20 9BX, United Kingdom

Interleukin 2 (IL2) has established immunotherapy as the fourth modality of cancer treatment. The clinical exploitation was greatly accelerated by the more widespread availability of the recombinant (rIL2) material. The design of the first clinical protocols with rIL2 was based on investigations in murine sarcomas of variable immunogenicity at the National Cancer Institute, Bethesda. Interest was stimulated in particular by 3 reports of objective responses in patients with refractory cancers treated with rIL2 with and without lymphokine activated killer (LAK) cells, [1-3]. The chronology of these early NCI and subsequent studies from other centres is shown in Table 1 with appropriate references, [4-51]. Since then, there has been a plethora of clinical and allied reports concerning rIL2. This review will briefly summarise some of the clinical aspects of rIL2 therapy when used alone (without LAK cells) and recent combinations of rIL2 with other materials.

Pharmacokinetics

The serum half-life is quite short with an alpha phase of 2 to 13 minutes and a slower beta elimination phase of 32 to 70 minutes after rIL2 bolus injection [8,15,52,53]. At the maximum tolerated dose (MTD) of 3000 U/kg/hour by continuous infusion of rIL2, serum levels of 5-10 U/ml and 137 U/ml at 2 hours after a bolus dose i.v of $3.8 \times 10^6 U/m^2$ were obtained [8, 53]. With a continuous infusion at the MTD of $3 \times 10^6 U/m^2/day$ for 7 days, the Wisconsin group found steady state values of approximately 30 U/ml [52]. Other studies by Thompson et al. in 1987 [12] showed that 2-hour i.v. infusions produced the highest peak levels but disappearance was rapid with a half-life of about 30 minutes. A 2-hour i.v. infusion and the same dose ($3 \times 10^6 U$) subcutaneously gave serum levels of 8-24 U/ml for 4-5 hours on i.v administration which were more prolonged, 8-10 hours after subcutaneous injection. Within 1 hour of stopping a 24-hour continuous i.v. infusion at the same dose, there was extremely rapid loss with low levels (3 U/ml) detectable in the serum. The steady state rIL2 level obtained with continuous infusion is known to be able to activate LAK cells *in vitro* [52]. Subcutaneous, intraperitoneal and intrapleural routes of rIL2 administration result in more prolonged half-lives than those obtained by i.v. bolus [12,14,30]. Detectable levels were reported for over 24 hours in pleural effusions and over 8 hours in the serum following intrapleural instillation [14]. The use of body cavities, the spleen and liver as reservoir sites to expand NK (natural killer) and LAK activity is of interest and the pharmacokinetics of rIL2 are obviously important in planning treatment regimens.

Although there are a number of recombinant IL2 preparations available, the most commonly used are those of the Cetus corporation and of Hoffmann-La Roche. For comparison purposes, one Cetus unit is approximately equivalant to 2.3 Hoffman-La Roche units and a standard biological response modifier programme (BRMP) rIL2 unit is equivalent to a Hoffmann-La Roche unit. This difference in activity should be considered when attempts are made to compare across studies in which different rIL2 preparations

Table 1. Overview of Interleukin 2 clinical trials in oncology

Year	Study	No. of patients entered	Findings	Reference and number
1980	Adopted transfer of long-term cultured peripheral blood lymphocytes (LAK cells)	3	Small cell numbers (less than 5×10^8) safely infused into patients	Lotze et al [4]
1983	Administration of natural (Jurkat-derived) IL2	16	Natural IL2 safely infused in patients at doses up to 2 mg	Mazumder et al [15]
1984	Adoptive transfer of LAK cells activated with rIL2	6	LAK cells activated with rIL2 could be safely infused into patients	Rosenberg et al [6]
1984	Intra and peri-lesional cancer	10	5CR and 4PR noted	Pizza et al [7]
1985	Administration of rIL2 alone: phase I study	20	Safe administration of rIL2, no tumour responses	Lotze et al [8]
1985	Administration of LAK cells and rIL2	25	Regression of metastatic cancer seen in 44% of patients	Rosenberg et al [1]
1986	Weekly bolus injection, phase I study	17	10^3-10^6U/m^2 no enhancement in cytotoxicity, no responses	Atkins et al [9]
1986	Administration of high dose bolus rIL2 alone iv or intraperitoneally	10	Regression of metastases in 3 melanomas	Lotze et al [10]
1986	Intraperitonal rIL2	7	Serum levels maintained up to 8 hours with increased NK activity 1 PR in hepatic + lung metastases	Lotze et al [11]
1987	Weekly 2hr, or 24hr iv or sc administration of rIL2	22	No responses bio-availability study	Thompson et al [12]
1987	Administration of rIL2 alone or with LAK cells	157	9CR and 20 PR (19% OR)	Rosenberg et al [2]
1987	Constant infusion of rIL2 with LAK cells	48	Less toxicity, 13 PR (27% OR)	West et al [3]
1987	Periodate rIL2 activated lymphocytes + rIL2 in renal cancer	13	6 PR (46% OR)	Wang et al [13]
1987	Intrapleural rIL2 in malignant effusions	11	Reduction in effusions and generation of LAK activity	Yasumoto et al [14]
1987	Bolus rIL2 in melanoma: phase I study	12	No responses Toxicity not severe	Marolda et al [15]
1987	Intravesicular IL2 +BCG in bladder cancer	13	Few side effects with BCG + rIL2 compared with BCG alone	Merguerian et al [16]

Table 1. Overview of Interleukin 2 clinical trials in oncology (continued)

Year	Study	No. of patients entered	Findings	Reference and number
1988	Administration rIL2 alone or with LAK cells	222	16CR and 26PR (19% OR) in various cancers	Rosenberg et al [17]
1988	Repeated 4 day cycles of continuous infusion of rIL2	11	1PR in renal cancer Little toxicity, marked immunomodulation	Sondel et al [18]
1988	Independent evaluation of rIL2 + LAK (Rosenberg protocol) in renal cancer by EWG	222	2CR and 3PR (16% OR) confirmed activity	Fisher et al [19]
1988	Continuous infusion rIL2, dose and duration study	23	No responses but continuous infusion. Greater immunomodulation and toxicity than bolus	Thompson et al [20]
1988	rIL2 with cyclophosphamide in melanoma	27	1CR, 5PR (22% OR)	Mitchell et al [21]
1988	Four weekly, 4 day infusions of rIL2 in melanoma and renal cancer	23	3 PR (13% OR)	Sosman et al [22]
1988	Weekly 24 hour infusions of rIL2 in melanoma and renal cancer	16	No responses, enhanced NK activity	Richards et al [23]
1988	Intralymphatic administration of IL2 and LAK cells	7	3PR and 4CR in various cancers	Pizza et al [24]
1988	Low dose rIL2, 3×10^4 U/kg and LAK	28	4CR + 9PR (46% OR) low toxicity	Schoof et al [25]
1988	rIL2 sc and bolus iv. with iv beta interferon	47	1PR (2% OR)	Krigel et al [26[
1988	rIL2 2hr iv. $3 \times 10^6 U/m^2/dx5$ in renal cancer	10	1CR and 2PR (33% OR)	Javadpour et al [27]
1988	Intratumoural (cavity) IL2 + with LAK in malignant brain tumours	23	6PR (26% OR) Improvement in symptoms	Yoshida et al [28]
1988	IL2 low dose perilymphatically in recurrent head and neck cancer	10	3CR + 3PR (60% OR)	Cortesina et al [29]
1988	Intraperitoneal rIL2 for advanced ovarian cancer	7	No responses. Outpatient tolerable dose 10×6 U/m^2	Chapman et al [30]
1988	LAK + rIL2 for recurrent glioblastoma. Treatment given intratumour cavity or via Ommaya reservoir.	13	No obvious survival benefit	Merchant et al [31]

Table 1. Overview of Interleukin 2 clinical trials in oncology (continued)

Year	Study	No. of patients entered	Findings	Reference and number
1989	LAK + rIL2 for hepato-cellular carcinoma	10	1PR (10% OR) No major side effects	Onishi et al [32]
1989	Phase I study rIL2 in children	7	No objective responders	Nasr et al [33]
1989	rIL2 + LAK 3×10^4U/kg 8 hourly iv bolus	26	3 PR in renal cell carcinoma and 1 PR in melanoma (15% OR). Toxicity greater if previous nephrectomy	Stahel et al [34]
1989	Low dose rIL2 iv and sc as OP 10^6U/d for 21-240 days in renal cancer	13	2CR and 1PR (23% OR)	Marumo et al [35]
1989	Low dose rIL2 iv as OP 1.5-3×10^6U/m^2 d1-5	35	3PR in 12 lymphoma patients (9% OR)	Allison et al [36]
1989	rIL2 sc with iv beta interferon	50	2PR (4% OR) MTDs identified for combination	Paolozzi et al [37]
1989	rIL2 alone or with TNF, alpha interferon, antibodies, cyclophosphamide, LAK cells, or TIL cells: NCI update	596	26CR and 78PR (17% OR) in various cancers	Rosenberg et al [38]
1989	Intrasplenic and intravenous bolus rIL2 in melanoma	31	4 PR (13 OR) Toxicity manageable despite high doses	Thatcher et al [39]
1989	rIL2+ LAK in melanoma Extramural Working Group	78	1CR and 11PR (15 % OR)	Sznol et al [40]
1989	rIL2+ dacarbazine in melanoma	27	2CR and 4PR (22 OR %)	Stoter et al [41]
1989	rIL2+ dacarbazine in melanoma	32	1 CR and 6 PR (22 OR%)	Flaherty et al [42]
1989	rIL2 + low dose cyclophos-phamide in melanoma and renal carcer	32	2 PR (6% OR)	Lindermann et al [43]
1989	rIL2 $\pm$ LAK $\pm$ doxorubicin	69	24 PR (35% OR) in various cancers	Paciucci et al [44]
1989	rIL2 + LAK Memphis update	114	2 CR and 19PR. (18% OR) in various cancers	West et al [45]
1989	rIL2 $\pm$ LAK cells in renal cancer	93	7CR and 13PR (21% OR)	Negrier et al [46]
1989	Continuous infusion, rIL2 in ovarian cancer: phase II study	11	1 CR pathologically confirmed at laparotomy	Panici et al [47]

Table 1. Overview of Interleukin 2 clinical trials in oncology (continued)

Year	Study	No. of patients entered	Findings	Reference and number
1989	rIL2, alpha interferon both iv phase II study	94	7 CR and 18PR (27% OR) in various cancers	Rosenberg et al [48]
1989	Continuous iv rIL2 and daily im alpha interferon	27	1CR and 6PR (26% OR) in various cancers	Lee et al [49]
1990	Intrasplenic and intravenous bolus rIL2 + flavone acetic acid in melanoma	34	4 PR and 1CR (15% OR)	Thatcher et al [50]
1990	High dose intermittent rIL2 in renal cancer	44	1CR and 4PR (11% OR)	Bukowski et al [51]

d - day   hr - hour   iv - intravenous, im - intramuscular, sc - subcutaneous
CR - Complete Response   PR - Partial Response   OR - Objective Response
OP - Out Patient   MTD - Maximum tolerated dose

are used. Occasionally, antibodies to rIL2 have been detected, almost invariably non-neutralising, and do not appear to be clinically important [9,53,54].

Immunomodulation

Major immunological changes occur following IL2 administration. These changes have been investigated almost entirely in the peripheral blood. It is difficult to summarise the changes because of wide variability in patient characteristics, rIL2 dosage, scheduling and sample timing. The immunological assays and parameters reported are also inconsistent, e.g., different target cells have been used for cytotoxicity assays, different methods of reporting results in terms either of cell percentages or of absolute cell numbers and different methods of expressing cytotoxicity in terms of total lytic units or on a per cell number basis.

Cell Number and Phenotype Changes

There is a consistent lymphopenia which occurs within a few hours of rIL2 administration. Recovery is usually seen 24-48 hours after bolus intravenous administration or the end-

ing of a continuous i.v. infusion. Recovery is immediately followed by a rebound and usually an over-shoot in most studies (see Table 2 for references, and [9, 62]). The changes in the lymphocyte count have been shown to be dose and schedule dependent in some studies [8,12,20,44,52,57] but not in all [58]. Constant infusion and twice-weekly schedules have been associated with a greater lymphocytosis [8,12,20,44,52,57]. A marked eosinophilia has also been frequently observed [18,22,23,39,55,57].

Some studies have examined the cell phenotype in the first few days of rIL2 treatment. Rapid loss of NK activity and LAK precursor cells (determined in assay systems containing in-vitro rIL2) within 5-15 minutes and lasting until recovery of the lymphocyte count, have been described. This loss is usually non-selective and includes both T and B cells and cells with the IL2 receptor [8,12,18,55,56]. However, Creekmore et al. noted T but no B cell loss [57]. The loss of lytic function (NK) and the reduction in proliferative response to rIL2 but not to PHA suggests loss of responsive cells within the circulation rather than suppression of any remaining cells [52]. These dynamic changes in the cell phenotype, like the changes in the actual lymphocyte count, have also been shown to be dose and schedule dependent [8,12,52,55,56]. The over-shoot in lymphocyte count can be as much as 10-16-fold with

Table 2. Enhanced immunomodulation of peripheral blood following IL2 alone

Investigator	Ref No.	Dose/U Schedule	Lympho-cytosis	Activated Phenotype	Circulating NK	LAK	OR
Lotze et al.	8	Cetus B, CIV 10^2-10^6/kg*	+	+	-	-	0/20
Thompson et al.	12	Hoffman-La Roche 2h,24h CIV, SC. once weekly every 2 wks x 4, 0.3-30x10^6*	-	-	-	-	0/22
Thompson et al.	20	Hoffman-La Roche 2h, 24h CIV daily x5 every 2 wks x 4 0.3x10^6, 3x10^6/m^2/d (also B, 8 h, 3x10^6/m^2/d)	+	+	+	+	1/23
Sosman et al.	22	Hoffman-La Roche B, CIV, B+CIV daily x4 every week x 4 1x10^6, 3x10^6/m^2/d	+	+	+	+	3/28
Richards et al.	23	Cetus 24h CIV weekly x 6 3.0 - 10.0x10^6/m^2/d	+	NT	+	-	0/16
Paciucci et al.	44	Cetus CIV daily x 6, weekly x4	+	+	+	+	13/32
Sano et al.	55	Shionogi 2h, 24h CIV daily x5, x28d 4 courses 0.33-2.2x10^6/m^2/d	+	+	+	+	0/34
Hank et al.	56	Hoffman-La Roche B, CIV, daily x7 10^3-10^7/m^2 or CIV daily x 4 1-3 10^6/m^2/d weekly x4	+	NT	+	+/-	0/25
Creekmore et al.	57	Hoffman-La Roche 24h, CIV weekly x4 then twice weekly x4 10^3-3x10^7/m^2/d	+	+	+	+	2/33
Ghosh et al.	58	Cetus B, x 5d/week every 3 weeks x 3 1 - 16.4x10^6/m^2	+	+	+	+	4/20

*Total dose B-Bolus, CIV-continuous infusion, SC-subcutaneous, NT-not tested, OR-objective response, d-day

continuous infusions and tends to be greater than with the 8-hourly i.v. bolus regimen [8,52,63].

The lymphocyte count rebound and the number of cells of certain phenotypes, e.g., those bearing the IL2 receptor and those exhibiting a proliferative response to rIL2, can be progressively enhanced by additional IL2 treatment cycles [18,22,39,56,58]. The enhancement is seen when the interval between treatment is only a few days, as in the Wisconsin studies, but not with more prolonged intervals [20,52,58]. The importance of the infusion duration was neatly described by the study of Thompson et al., 1988 [20]. Lymphocytosis induced by 3×10^5 U/m^2/d infused over 24 hours was significantly higher than that induced by 3×10^6 U/m^2/d given over 2 hours also for 5 consecutive days. These data indicate that, for equal doses, continuous infusion had a greater biological effect. The lymphocyte rebound is associated with increased numbers of "activated" cells with NK, LAK (precursor and effector) function and of cells expressing the IL2 receptor, class II MHC antigens and markers for killer activity [20,22,52,55,56,58,63]. The changes in cell phenotype again appear to be dose and schedule dependent [20,22,52,57]. The increase seen in some phenotypes, e.g., IL2 receptor-bearing cells, suggests preferential activation of certain subsets and a relative lack of effect on B cells [20,22]. However, the representation of these cells is not consistent, there was no increase in IL2 receptor bearing cells in the Creekmore study [57], suggesting that the presence of this cell type was not essential for the enhanced lytic activity observed.

Lytic Activity

Arguably the most important feature of rIL2 immunomodulation is the potential increase in cytotoxicity. Although killer cell activity (NK) against the K562 cell line is regularly induced and increased, LAK activity is less frequently observed (see Table 2). Some studies have failed to demonstrate either LAK precursor (LAKp) and more often LAK effector (LAKe) activity [8,9,12,23]. Other studies have shown induction of NK and particularly LAK activity

in peripheral blood of patients in whom such activity was previously absent [20,22,55-60,64]. Thompson et al. [20] reported that two-thirds of patients developed LAK activity which was dose dependent, however, Ghosh et al. [58], who also demonstrated increased LAK activity in 9 of 20 patients investigated comprehensively, were not able to show dose dependence. In general, NK and LAK activity appear to be induced and enhanced more reliably with continuous infusion and higher doses than by other schedules or lower doses. The differences in lytic activity reported in various studies may of course be more a feature of sample timing with a failure of detection rather than a failure of induction of killer activity [12]. Although other studies, e.g., Ghosh, 1989 [58], indicate that only a proportion of patients will respond with LAK enhancement and this enhancement is not dependent on the prior presence of LAK precursor cells, LAK activity in this study was unlikely to have been missed as blood was sampled several times per week.

The onset of increased killer activity has been determined in only a few studies in which frequent daily sampling was undertaken (see Table 3). Information on the duration of any enhanced cytotoxicity is also sparse. Several reports indicate that increased cytotoxicity lasts only 7-10 days after finishing IL2 treatment [18,58]. Elevated NK but not LAK activity has been noted for 35-42 days [44,55] and up to 180 days by Walewski et al. [61] with continuous infusions of rIL2.

The increase in NK and LAK activity, even when it occurs, is quite modest, with only several-fold increase over the pre-IL2 baseline values (see Table 3). If the lymphocytosis is also taken into consideration, the cytotoxic potential can increase 40-300 fold over pre-IL2 levels despite only modest increases of about 10-fold in lytic activity [22]. Additional rIL2 treatment cycles have progressively increased NK and LAK activity, which was significantly greater after 4, weekly cycles than after the first [22]. Progressive augmentation of activity was also noted following continuous infusion for 6 days of each week for 4 weeks by Paciucci et al. [44]. This progressive enhancement presumably results from augmentation of residual increases in lytic activity, providing that the interval between rIL2 cycles is not too long. Boosting NK and

Table 3. Onset of enhanced NK LAK activity in peripheral blood with the maximum increase following IL2 alone

Investigator	Ref.	NK		LAKp		LAKe	
		Onset	Maximum Increase	Onset	Maximum Increase	Onset	Maximum Increase
Lotze et al. 1985	[8]	1-2d	4x	2-4d	200x	0	0
Thompson et al. 1987	[12]	0	0	0	0	0	0
Sondel et al. 1988	[18]	NT	NT	5d	20x	5d	7x
Thompson et al. 1988	[20]	7-10d	8x	6d	60x	6d	0-48 LU (No pt. had LAK activity pre IL2)
Sosman et al. 1988	[22]	28d	5x	28d	22x	28d	8x
Richards et al. 1988	[23]	14d	14x	NT	NT	0	0
Sano et al. 1988	[55]	1-5d	3x	NT	NT	3-5d	3x
Hank et al. 1988	[56]	6d	2x	1d	15x	1d	5x
Creekmore et al. 1989	[57]	28d	5x	NT	NT	28d	11x
Ghosh et al. 1989	[58]	7-8d	4x	7-8d	0	7-8d	5x
McMannis et al. 1988	[59]	NT	40x	NT	NT	4-6wks	0-25 LU (no pt. had LAK activity pre IL2)
Gambacorti-Passerini 1989	[60]	4d	2x	0	0	4d	3x
Walewski 1989	[61]	4-9d	2x	NT	NT	4-9d	4x

NK, natural killer activity; LAKp, lymphokine-activated killer precursor activity; LAKe, lymphokine-activated killer effector activity; LU, lytic units; NT, not tested

LAK activity following systemic intravenous rIL2 has been obtained by adding more rIL2 to the *in vitro* cytotoxicity assay system [56]. This type of experiment and others suggest that NK and LAK activity is dependent on the continued presence of IL2 for enhancement and that IL2 "starvation" may be responsible for the rapid decline in peripheral blood ac-tivity [52]. Attention to scheduling and dosage should help the design of protocols and pro-mote greater enhancement of cytotoxicity *in vivo*. Such protocols should thereby reduce the need for *ex vivo* LAK cell generation.
The release of other cytokines, including gamma interferon, tumour necrosis factor, etc. is also promoted by rIL2 and can be detected

in the serum of some patients [65-67]. Although these secondary cytokines could well have important antitumour effects and be responsible for some of the toxicity, there is also recent evidence that gamma interferon may exert an inhibitory interaction [68]. Furthermore, increasing the number of IL2 receptor-bearing cells and/or soluble receptor may conceivably remove or reduce lytic activity, the receptors binding the rIL2 administered.

Future studies of rIL2 therapy should then assess the correlation, if any, between circulating killer activity and cytokine levels with toxicity and antitumour effect. Tumour biopsy material should be appropriately used or stored to determine more directly the effects of rIL2 therapy; investigations which, sadly, in the most part are still lacking.

Toxicity

The first clinical trials from the Surgery Branch of the NCI reported considerable multisystem toxicity (see Table 4). The review by Lee et al. of 317 patients who were treated with 423 courses of rIL2 with or without LAK cells or cyclophosphamide, highlighted the cardio-respiratory toxicity [69]. Hypotension was the most frequent major problem requiring pressors and i.v. fluid in 65% of patients. Severe dyspnoea occurred in 9% of patients and 6% required intubation. Pleural effusions, ascites and severe peripheral oedema occurred in less than 4% of patients, but with significant weight gain (> than 10% of body weight) in 32% of the patients. Angina and signs of myocardial ischaemia were noted in 3% and myocardial infarction in 1%. It should be emphasised that this patient population had been given multiple daily bolus doses at the maximum tolerated level (10^5U/kg). In a more recent update of 155 patients treated with 236 courses of IL2 alone, there were 4 (less than 3%) treatment-related deaths, which compares very favourably with current intensive therapy given for chemosensitive tumours [38].

Cumulative cardiovascular disturbance is the major dose-limiting toxicity, the features resemble those seen in septicaemic shock and arise from a capillary leak syndrome.

Reduction in systemic vascular resistance, tachycardia, hypotension with loss of albumin into the extravascular space are the main features. The associated intravascular volume depletion leads to oliguria, marked sodium retention and increase in serum urea and creatinine. High levels of endothelial leukocyte and intercellular, adhesion molecules are represented diffusely on the endothelium of skin biopsies of rIL2 patients, and are not confined, as normally, to specific inflammatory sites [70]. These endothelial changes with resulting leakage of macromolecules are likely to be mediated by TNF and other cytokines and it is known that killer cell activity is also required for this leak syndrome. Meir et al. [71] have indicated that TNF and other cytokines can in certain experimental situations diminish LAK cell-induced capillary leak, so the aetiology of the syndrome is still unclear.

Elevated cardiac enzymes, cardiac arrhythmias, ischaemia etc. are probably due a toxic myocarditis, but only rarely have cardiac deaths been reported [69]. Respiratory distress, sometimes severe, is caused by pulmonary oedema and capillary leakage, cardiac toxicity and possibly, in some circumstances, by fluid overload given in an attempt to restore blood pressure. Neuropsychiatric side effects can also occur, but coma is now recognised to be usually due to the presence of pre-existing CNS metastatic disease. The presence of CNS metastases is a contraindication to systemic rIL2 therapy. More common side effects include fever, chills and general lethargy with a 'flu-like' illness lasting for a few days.

Despite the wide spectrum of possible side effects, seen principally with the daily high-dose bolus therapy, the vast majority of patients are able to leave hospital 1 to 3 days after completion of even these most taxing treatment regimens. There also has been an increase in some patients' Karnofsky performance scores with rIL2 treatment even at high dose [39,50]. Only one possible exacerbation of tumour growth (Kaposi's sarcoma) has been reported with a combination of rIL2 and beta interferon [72]. Transient volume increases occasionally have been noted in tumours, probably due to local inflammatory reaction; again, there is a rapid improvement on completion of rIL2 therapy.

Table 4. Toxicities of Interleukin 2 treatment

	DESCRIPTION	COMMENTS
Systemic	Chills, fever	Induction of IL2, IFN gamma, possibly IL6
Cardiopulmonary	Capillary leak syndrome Fluid shifts Hypotension Oedema Effusions etc.	
	Decreased systemic vascular resistance Increased cardiac output Decreased arterial pressure	Pathophysiology similar to gram negative sepsis - possibly related to TNF and IFN-gamma induction
	Angina Arrhythmias Myocardial infarction/myocarditis	
	Dyspnoea Pulmonary oedema	
Renal	Oliguria	Largely pre-renal
Gastrointestinal	Anorexia Nausea and vomiting Diarrhoea Stomatitis Increased bilirubin Elevated transaminases	TNF (cachectin) related Intra-hepatic cholestasis
Neuropsychiatric	Lethargy Hallucinations delusions, disorientation Stupor, coma (in assocation with brain metastases)	Worsening of cerebral oedema
Haematological	Anaemia Thrombocytopenia Lymphopenia during IL2 administration Rebound lymphocytosis following cessation of IL2 Eosinophilia Abnormal coagulation	Suppression of bone marrow Unclear ? Redistribution ? IL5 related
Endocrinological	Increased cortisol Increased prolactin Increased growth hormone hypothyroidism	Appears to be self-limiting; ? exacerbation of underlying autoimmune thyroiditis
Dermatological	Diffuse macular erythema Pruritic rash Dry skin Desquamation	Biopsy nonspecific
Miscellaneous	Catheter sepsis	

Modified from Parkinson 1988 [67]

Methods to Decrease Toxicity

Although there is a wide variety of side effects, these are predictable and with experienced staff can be minimised. Recently, outpatient administration of rIL2 has become possible [35,36,73]. Toxicity is dose and schedule dependent but the relationship is difficult to interpret as most reports only give the intended protocol dose rather than the actual dose of rIL2 administered. In general, continuous i.v. infusion over several days or bolus high-dose therapy on alternate days is better tolerated than daily high-dose bolus treatment [39,50,52]. The high doses used by the NCI group were based on murine sarcoma studies and curative results in experimental models can now be obtained by lower doses [74]. Another advantage of the continuous infusion is that it allows interruption if side effects do develop, with restart or discontinuation of the infusion as appropriate. Contradicting this general experience was the study of Thompson et al. [20]. Two-hour i.v. or bolus doses over 15 minutes were compared with 24-hour infusions at the same total dose. It was noted, in fact, that the toxicity was greater for the 24-hour infusion. This study illustrates the difficulties of dose and schedule interpretations. Ibuprofen has been shown to be effective in reducing the pyrexia and has a marked benefit on symptom scores as shown by the study of Eberlein et al. [75]. In this study, no significant difference in response rate or in immunomodulation was found when ibuprofen was used. Indomethacin should not be used as it reduces intrarenal prostaglandin production, which is an important mediator of renal blood flow autoregulation. Indomethacin may therefore compound renal toxicity following a hypotensive episode. Steroids can be used if severe toxicity occurs but should not be used prophylactically as they diminish the effectiveness of rIL2 [76]. Paracetamol is also of value in reducing the pyrexia, chills and 'flulike' symptoms and can be given regularly. Previous nephrectomy for hypernephroma does not, in itself, give a greater risk of renal toxicity for patients on rIL2 [77]. The most important risk factor for renal toxicity was the baseline serum creatinine; if this was normal, there was no difference for patients with hypernephroma who had had a nephrectomy and others with intact kidneys.

The most important aspect of the care of patients receiving rIL2 is good nursing and medical practice by a team experienced in the clinical use of rIL2. Such organisation not only gives the patient confidence but also facilitates the prevention and reduction of side effects through prompt and appropriate intervention. The previous requirement for regular access to intensive care facilities for patients treated with rIL2 is now no longer necessary [39,50,52].

Tumour Response

rIL2 Alone

Recombinant IL2, when used alone, certainly has anticancer activity in humans. The earlier dose-ranging Phase I/II studies were performed in patients who were deliberately selected on the basis of having failed previous anticancer therapies or when no standard treatment was available. These patients had resistant cancers: malignant melanoma, renal carcinoma, sarcoma, malignant lymphoma and adenocarcinomas from a variety of sites: colon, lung, breast etc. Not surprisingly, given the nature of this patient population, dosage regimen and short treatment times, only 2 responses were observed in 199 patients (see Table 2 and [8,9,12,15,23,33,55,57,81,82]). Despite these disadvantages, disease was stabilised in some patients [9,12]. Lotze et al. in 1986 were the first to report tumour responses (although partial) in 3 of 6 melanoma patients who had received high-dose bolus rIL2 [10]. Subsequently, a number of reports of i.v. rIL2 alone have confirmed activity, principally in metastatic renal cell carcinoma and malignant melanoma (see Table 5). In the Rosenberg update, which describes the largest series, i.e., 155 patients treated with i.v. high-dose bolus rIL2 alone, there was a 22% response rate (4 complete, CR and 8 partial, PR) in 54 patients with renal cancer and a 24% response rate (10 PR) in 42 patients with melanoma [38]. If the studies in Table 5, which summarises the larger series, are considered, there is a 16% re-

Table 5. Clinical responses with rIL2 alone in phase II studies of more than 10 patients

Investigator	Ref.	Dose (U) Schedule	Renal	Melanoma (responses/patients entered)	Lymphoma	Colon
Sondel et al.	[18]	1 or $3\times10^6/m^2$ CIV daily x4 each wk x4	1/6	0/5	-	-
Thompson et al.	[20]	3×10^5 or $3\times10^6/m^2$ 2h or 24h CIV daily x5 every 2wks x4 (also B, 8h, $3\times10^6/m^2$)	0/5	0/15	-	0/6
Sosman et al.	[22]	1 or $3\times10^6/m^2$ B, CIV, B+ CIV daily x4 each wk x4	3/21	0/7	-	-
Marumo et al.	[35]	10^{6*} daily iv or sc for 21-240 days	3/13	-	-	-
Allison et al.	[36]	1.5 or $3.0\times10^6/m^2$ B, d1-5 every 2 wks x4	0/2	0/8	3/9	0/6
Rosenberg et al.	[38]	10^5/kg or $1-6\times10^6/m^2$ tds, d1-5, repeating after 7-10d	12/54	10/42	0/11	0/12
Thatcher et al.	[39]	$1-16.4\times10^6/m^2$ B, d1,3,5,7 every 3 wk x3	-	4/31	-	-
Paciucci et al.	[44]	$3.4\times10^6/m^2$/d CIV, daily x6 weekly x4	1/6	6/7	1/3	2/7
Negrier et al.	[46]	$3\times10^6/m^2$/d CIV d1-5, 12-17 repeat d35	6/42	-	-	-
Bukowski et al.	[51]	$10^7/m^2$, B 3 times weekly	5/44	-	-	-
Javadpour et al.	[78]	$3\times10^6/m^2$/d 2h, d1-5 every 2 wks x8	3/15	-	-	-

CIV, continuous iv infusion; B, Bolus iv; wk, week; d, day; h, hour; *total dose; tds, three times per day

sponse rate for renal cancer (34/208) with 10 CR and 24 PR and a 17% response rate for melanoma (20/115) with 20 PR and no CR. The response rate for malignant lymphoma is 13% and for colon cancer 6% (see Table 5). Allison et al. reported activity in chronic lymphocytic leukaemia and their treatment schedule could be given on an out-patient basis [36]. Activity in B-chronic lymphocytic leukaemia has also been reported [83].

Local-Regional IL2

Local-regional IL2 has a number of possible advantages. It should give higher concentrations of IL2 at the site of tumour and diminish the toxicity seen with systemic therapy. These and other advantages are more fully described by Roth and Kirkwood [84]. Surprisingly, only a few clinical trials with local-regional IL2 have been reported. The first was the intra-lesional and peri-lesional use of lymphoblastoid IL2 by Pizza et al. in 10 patients with advanced bladder tumour. Of these patients, 4 underwent CR, 2 PR following IL2, given on 2 or 3 occasions over 7-54 days [7]. A further update of this report showed similar results in 14 patients [85]. Another study in 5 patients with advanced T4 bladder cancer used high-dose continuous bladder perfusions over 5 days. The total dose of IL2 over the 5 days was 15×10^6 units. Again, there were no significant side effects but eosinophilia was marked with one complete response [86]. A combination of intra-vesicular rIL2 and BCG has also been investigated by Merguerian et al. in 13 patients with resected transitional cell carcinoma of the bladder. The rIL2 was given with BCG and there was an 85% disease-free survival of 6-24 months. It was considered that the combination was possibly superior to full conventional dose of BCG alone, in terms of side effects and efficacy [16].

The intra-pleural use of rIL2 in 11 patients with malignant pleurisy has already been commented upon [14]. In 9 of these 11 patients, there was disappearance of the effusion and cancer cells occurring 4 to 10 days after the start of the treatment. Fever and eosinophilia were the main side effects, the patients' survival ranged from 7-21 months. A similar study reported in abstract form confirmed the feasibility of using intra-pleural followed by continuous i.v. infusions of rIL2 in mesothelioma and adenocarcinoma of the lung [87].

Local injection of rIL2 was reported by Cortesina et al., based on experimental models devised by Forni. Ten patients with advanced head and neck carcinoma received low-dose Jurkatt IL2 (200 units only) injected peri-lymphatically close to the mastoid. Six patients with bilateral and contralateral neck nodes underwent response with 3 CRs lasting for up to 6 months. There were no systemic disturbances with this low-dose treatment [29].

The most frequent use of regional IL2 is by the intra-peritoneal route. This was originally investigated by Lotze et al. in 7 patients with melanoma, ovarian carcinoma or colorectal carcinoma. The rIL2 was given via a Tenckhoff catheter as bolus doses 3 times a day. There were considerable constitutional side effects, but one patient with melanoma

had marked response in pulmonary and hepatic metastases. However, treatment was complicated by the presence of dense adhesions and bulky tumour which restricted the intra-peritoneal access [11]. Chapman et al. also used the intra-peritoneal route with escalating dosages in 7 patients with ovarian malignancy. Again, this was associated with some systemic toxicity but no major hypotension. No responses were seen, but the dose of $10^6 U/m^2$ was well tolerated and could be given twice weekly to outpatients [30].

It is clear from these studies that rIL2 can be given in a local-regional fashion with activation of the immune system, and tumour responses have been seen. Combinations of intra-lymphatic and intra-lesional IL2 have been investigated, see Table 1 and [24,32, 84]. The use of intra-lesional rIL2 (into the tumour cavity or via an Ommaya reservoir) with LAK cells has been reported for malignant brain tumours [28,31].

rIL2 and Chemotherapy

Low-dose cyclophosphamide ($350mg/m^2$ i.v.) was used by Mitchell et al. to decrease suppressor T cells before rIL2 treatment, thereby possibly enhancing tumour response and reducing the toxicity due to "immune activation" [21]. In the 27 patients with disseminated melanoma, there was a 22% response rate (1 CR and 5 PR) with minor responses in another 8 patients. Interestingly, the rIL2 was given to outpatients over 15 minutes ($3.6 \times 10^6 U/m^2$) daily for 5 days in 2 successive weeks, starting 3 days after the cyclophosphamide. The dose-ranging Phase I study of Kolitz et al. using subcutaneous rIL2 and cyclophosphamide reported no responses in 18 patients with advanced malignancy [88]. However, in the multicentre German study with rIL2 ($3 \times 10^6 U/m^2/d$) given as a 30-minute i.v. infusion for 14 days, starting 3 days after cyclophosphamide, 2 responses (PR) in 18 patients with melanoma were noted (11%), although no patient with renal cancer responded [43].

The only other agent that has been evaluated in several studies is dacarbazine in melanoma. The study by Flaherty used a 24-hour infusion of DTIC ($1g/m^2$) every 4 weeks on day 1 with bolus doses of rIL2 (2-

$4 \times 10^6 U/m^2$) on days 15-19, 22-26. Although toxicity was considerable (dose-limiting fatigue 61% and hypotension 43% of patients), there was an objective response rate of 22% with 1 CR and 6 PR, in the study group of 32 patients [42]. Dacarbazine at lower dose ($850 mg/m^2$) has been given after continuous infusion (days 1-5, 11-17), rIL2, on day 26 [89]. There was a response rate of 22% in 27 patients (2 CR and 4 PR). The multicentre study by Shiloni et al. used the same dose of DTIC but followed by rIL2. In 30 melanoma patients, the objective response rate was 13% (2 CR and 2 PR) [90].

Doxorubicin (30 mg/m²) has been used with a continuous infusion of rIL2 in 12 patients with non-small-cell lung cancer and breast carcinoma. Three partial and 2 minor responses were observed [44]. The other agent currently being used in a number of colorectal studies is 5-fluorouracil, but data are too preliminary for comment. Combination chemotherapy, cisplatin and dacarbazine with rIL2 has given a 40% response rate in advanced melanoma (Flaherty, personal communication). Flavone acetic acid (FAA), a synthetic flavonoid, is known to act synergistically with rIL2 in curing murine tumours, either agent alone being ineffective. FAA will also enhance NK activity in patients about 24 hours after administration. These properties prompted the Manchester group to give FAA ($4.8 G/m^2$) 24 hours before high-dose bolus rIL2 ($11 \times 10^6 U/m^2$). In a group of 34 progressing melanoma patients with metastases in multiple organ sites, there was a response rate of 15% (1 CR and 4 PR) [50].

rIL2 with Other, Biological Agents

Synergism, upregulation of IL2 receptors on cytolytic effector cells, Fc receptors on IL2-activated cells and MHC class 1 expression on tumour cells, make combinations of rIL2 with Tumour Necrosis Factor (TNF), monoclonal antibodies and interferons therapeutically attractive.

Most clinical studies are still preliminary. In the NCI Phase I investigation, TNF (50-350 µg/m²) was given i.v. daily for 3 days followed by bolus 8-hourly rIL2 (3×10^4-$10^5 U/kg$), the sequence being synergistic in animal models. In 38 patients, there was a response rate of 10% (1 CR and 3 PR) in melanoma and renal cancer patients [38]. A subpopulation of IL2-activated cells bear Fc receptors which are capable of mediating antibody-dependent directed cytotoxicity. A rationale then exists for IL2-monoclonal antibody combinations. Preliminary studies are underway at the MD Anderson Hospital in Houston, but the NCI group found no responses in 12 melanoma and 20 colorectal patients [38].

It has been the alpha interferon and rIL2 combinations that have shown most promise [48,49]. In the MD Anderson study, 27 metastatic cancer patients were given rIL2 by continuous i.v. infusion ($1-3 \times 10^6 U/m^2/d$) for 4 days each week for 4 weeks. Courses were repeated after 2-4 weeks rest. Alpha interferon ($2-10 \times 10^6 U/m^2/d$) was given concurrently intramuscularly on the same days as rIL2. There were 1 complete and 3 partial responses, all in melanoma, out of a total of 10 patients with this tumour [49]. Side effects were described as manageable. The other recent study from the NCI was of 94 patients with metastatic cancer. Intravenous alpha interferon (3 or $6 \times 10^6 U/m^2$) was given shortly after 15-minute i.v. bolus doses every 8 hours of rIL2 ($1-4.5 \times 10^6 U/m^2$). Daily treatments were given for 5 consecutive days and repeated after 10 days rest. There was an overall 27% response rate for the total study group, with 3 CR an 10 PR in 39 melanoma patients and 4 CR and 7 PR in 35 renal cancer patients. A further partial response occurred in 1 of 9 patients with colorectal cancer [48]. The response rate appeared related to the dose used. No unexpected toxicity occurred, although there was one treatment-related death in this advanced patient population with resistant cancer.

The combination of subcutaneous and (later i.v.) rIL2 and i.v. beta interferon was examined by Krigel et al. in a Phase I study [26]. In 47 patients, there was one partial response (melanoma) in a schedule in which the cytokines were given by bolus dosing 3 times a week for 4 weeks. The dose-limiting toxicity was profound fatigue, depression, anorexia, weight loss and arthralgia rather than the toxicity from the capillary leak syndrome [26]. The other Phase I i.v. beta interferon study with rIL2 was of 50 patients in which 2, 1 patient with rectal cancer and 1 with bladder cancer, had partial responses [37]. These results are somewhat disappointing given beta interferon's marked tumourcidal activity in experimental systems. Gamma inteferon has also been used with rIL2 in a Phase I study by Wagstaff et al., but no tumour response data were reported [91].

Response Characteristics and Predictors

Objective tumour responses have been consistently recorded following rIL2 therapy. Most data concern metastatic malignant melanoma and renal cancer, as patients with these resistant malignancies are particularly suited for IL2 and other novel treatment programmes. In these cancers, the most frequent response sites are in lung, skin, subcutaneous areas and peripheral adenopathy [18,22,35,38,39,41-44,46,48-51,89,90]. Other non-visceral sites also respond, liver, intra-abdominal adenopathy and soft tissues, adrenal, mediastinal adenopathy, effusions. In some cases, these responses are complete [14,21,35,38,39,41,42,44,46,48-51,87, 89,90]. In the Negrier study, 19 responses occurred in lung versus 30 in all other sites. In this study, 10 regressions in primary renal tumours were also observed [46]. Complete responses have been reported more often in renal cell carcinoma than in melanoma.

Most responses are observed within the first 2 cycles of treatment, i.e., within 1-3 months [46,90]. Interestingly though, responses can evolve over several months. Patients with stable disease can convert to partial response and even to complete response, a process which can take 3-6 months, either whilst treatment is continuing or even after cessation of treatment [10,21,39,46,49]. Bukowski et al. found the median time to response was 49 days and varied between 19 and 115 days with a weekly rIL2 regimen [51]. Although Rosenberg et al. have observed only a few mixed responses and indicated that, if response occurred in one site, responses usually occurred in other sites as well, this observation has not been confirmed by others [21,38,39,49,50].

The responses that are obtained are not triv-

ial. Durable responses of several years have now been recorded with unmaintained remissions of up to 41 months in about 10% of the patients with metastatic melanoma and renal cancer [38, Thatcher, personal communication]. These durable remissions have occurred also in visceral sites such as the liver and lungs. In the largest series of Rosenberg et al., the durability of complete remissions in renal cancer after IL2 alone lasted from 25-34 months. The range for partial response duration, without progression, is somewhat wider: 3-27 months for renal cancer and 2-41 months for melanoma [38]. Other studies also have reported unmaintained remissions of over a year and in some cases 2 years [21,39,42,44,48,50,51,89]. There is now the potential for durable complete and partial remissions being produced by rIL2, even in patients with advanced tumour burdens.

Another important feature of rIL2 therapy is the stabilisation of previously progressing disease [39,50]. Patients with previously advanced progressing tumours who have undergone durable responses or had their disease stabilised also improve in terms of activity and performance status [21,38,39,48, 50]. Indeed, the duration of stabilisation can be very similar to that of objective remission in some series [37,89,90]. Nevertheless, the median duration of response is still quite short. For metastatic melanoma, it is of the order of 4-6 months [39,42,48,90]. The median duration of response for renal carcinoma tends to be slightly longer, 6 and 10 months [46,48]. Intriguingly, there is also the possibility that response to subsequent chemotherapy after rIL2 relapse may also be improved [39,50,83].

Survival data are still sparse, which is not suprising given the only recent implementation of rIL2 treatment. The median survival for these patients with advanced tumours ranges from 8-13 months for melanoma [39,50, 89] and 9-11 months for renal cancer [46,51]. Nevertheless, it is now clear that a proportion of patients with advanced and resistant tumours are exhibiting substantial antitumour effects and symptom palliation with rIL2 treatment. The benefit in some continues for many months and occasionally for years after end of treatment with rIL2.

Response Predictors

There is no substantial evidence that any clinical, haematological or immunological parameter correlates significantly with tumour response or patient survival. Immunomodulation and, in particular, generation of LAK and NK activity show no consistent relationship with tumour response (see Table 2). There are 3 studies in which immunomodulation has been linked possibly with tumour response. Creekmore et al. in 1989 noted that 2 of 6 melanoma patients treated at a higher dose had partial responses and greater immune modulation was also seen at the higher (total) dosages, although dose intensity in this study may also have been important [57]. The 2 partial responders, however, did not differ significantly from other patients in terms of killer cell activity or rebound lymphocytosis, although they did have the 2 highest peak, eosinophil counts. The second study was that of Paciucci et al. using continuous infusion of rIL2. Again, tumour regression appeared to be related to rIL2 dose, but peak LAK activity after the first week of treatment was the only other parameter with a possible response correlation [44]. The only other study in which response appeared to be particularly related to cytotoxicity was that of Yasumoto et al. in 1987. Patients who responded to the intrapleural instillation of rIL2 also had induction of LAK activity compared with non-responders [14]. Cytotoxicity in general, however, has shown no significant difference between responders and non-responders. Eosinophilia is often very pronounced with rIL2 and could be of interest as eosinophils have potent activity. To date, correlation of tumour response and lymphocytosis has only been considered and in most series is not significant (see Table 2).

Dose and scheduling could be important in determining response. It has been suggested that continuous infusion (associated with tumour responses) was superior to bolus treatment where no responses were noted [20]. However, the dose relationship is unclear, and responses have been seen at lower rather than at the higher doses in some studies [36]. The dose-response relationship is difficult to interpret because dose reduction due to toxicity is rarely documented. Longer duration therapy but at lower doses may allow a longer interaction time between rIL2 and effector cells, with the possibility of obtaining a higher response rate. Nevertheless, a series of reports indicate that objective responses were more frequently observed at higher than at lower doses [22,38,44,46,48,49]. The situation remains complex, however, as the patients who respond are those who best tolerate the treatment and may in turn be most likely, biologically, to benefit from the higher doses possible in these individual patients [43].

One of the few comprehensive studies involved 93 patients from 6 different medical centres. A standard clinical and laboratory protocol was employed, with rIL2 and LAK cell transfusions [62]. Neither tumour reduction nor clinical toxicity correlated with rIL2 dose, cytolytic activity or with any other laboratory parameter in this study of melanoma, renal and colon cancer patients. There was a trend for subjects with the highest rebound lymphocytosis to have a tumour response. This trend supports the original suggestion by West et al. that a rebound lymphocytosis of $6,000/\mu l$ or greater was more often associated with tumour response than lower rebound counts [3], but is not confirmed by other studies (see Table 2). In another analysis of 95 patients with metastatic renal cell carcinoma treated with rIL2 with and without LAK cells, several parameters were also investigated [46]. Rebound lymphocytosis $(>7,000/\mu l)$, age, performance status, interval between diagnosis and treatment and the interval between primary diagnosis and occurrence of metastases were not significantly correlated with response [46]. Most studies have been performed in patients with chemotherapy-resistant tumours. Renal cell carcinoma and malignant melanoma particularly have been studied and it is in these tumours that most responses have been seen. Whether response to rIL2 in these 2 tumour types is a biological treatment feature or just circumstantial and a feature of the patient eligibility for these trials, is not clear.

The immunological mechanisms associated with tumour response may vary in different tumour types. The role of T cell-mediated mechanisms may be more important in melanoma response than renal cell carcinoma [67]. The only study in which tumour material was investigated [79] showed that patients treated with rIL2 and LAK therapy had evidence of T-cell proliferation and extensive lymphoid infiltrates in melanoma metastases from responding patients but not from non-responders or before treatment was instituted. These features in tumour biopsies from patients responding to rIL2 indicated that MHC-restricted T lymphocytes rather than LAK cells could be more important in melanoma. Interestingly, skin biopsies taken from the patients before rIL2 had only a small number of HLA-DR positive cells identified by immunochemistry, but the number markedly increased following treatment, changes that may be important in the development of an antitumour effect [79].

In conjunction with the role of T cell-mediated mechanisms in certain tumours, the relationship in melanoma patients of pre-existing thyroid antiboides and response is also interesting [67]. Hypothyroidism can follow treatment with rIL2 and LAK cells or just IL2 alone, possibly by exacerbating pre-existing autoimmune thyroiditis. Five out of 7 patients with hypothyroidism, but only 5 of 27 euthyroid patients had evidence of melanoma regression, indicating that the previous immunological status of the patient may be important in determining response [80]. Other mechanisms determining response would include plasma factors affecting the IL2-induced cytotoxicity, accessibility of cytolytic cells to the tumour and the tumour's inherent immunogenicity [67].

Future Prospects

Recombinant interleukin 2 has demonstrated significant activity in cancer patients who were previously resistant to all available treatment modalities. The optimal treatment regimen is still unknown, although methods aimed at reducing toxicity have already been successful. Patients can now be treated on a general oncology ward without the mandatory requirement for intensive care facilities. Other approaches to treatment administration, i.e., subcutaneous use, ambulatory pump infusions etc., may allow more prolonged exposure to rIL2 with better development of cytotoxicity and antitumour activity. Combinations of rIL2 with chemotherapy are already being intensively evaluated as are other combinations of rIL2 with cytolytic cells (LAK and TIL) described elsewhere.

Of particular interest are the 2 recent reports on the use of interleukin 2 with alpha-interferon and the obvious antitumour effect of this combination. To augment the cytolytic potential engendered by rIL2, other cytokines, e.g., GM-CSF, IL4, IL5, may have an important clinical role. Appropriate Phase I and Phase II data, therefore, are awaited with interest. Methods to reduce patients' response to the foreign protein of zenogenic monoclonal antibodies include "humanisation" or the use of high doses but brief exposures followed by prolonged rIL2, in order to maintain the previously activated effector cell function. Heteroaggregates containing anti CD-3 antibodies cross-linked to anti-target cell antibodies could allow more specific activity and increased tumour cell kill by CD-3 bearing cells, which tend to have little LAK activity. The use of rIL2 as an adjuvant in tumour vaccine therapy and to induce killer cells for leukaemia treatment and bone marrow purging are other possible developments.

The overriding requirement for developing optimal treatments with rIL2 either alone or in combination with other agents is the close and continuing collaboration between clinical oncologists and basic scientists. This collaboration has already given cancer medicine a new opportunity in rIL2 to treat previously resistant malignancies.

REFERENCES

1   Rosenburg SA, Lotze MT, Muul LM et al: Special report - Observations on the systemic administration of autologous lymphokine-activated killer cells and recombinant interleukin-2 to patients with metastatic cancer. N Engl J Med 1985 (313):1485-1492

2   Rosenberg SA, Lotze MT, Muul LM et al: A progress report on the treatment of 157 patients with advanced cancer using lymphokine-activated killer cells and interleukin-2 or high-dose interleukin-2 alone. N Engl J Med 1987 (316):889-897

3   West WH, Tauer KW, Yannelli JR et al: Constant-infusion recombinant interleukin-2 in adoptive immunotherapy of advanced cancer. N Engl J Med 1987 (316):898-905

4   Lotze MT, Line BR, Mathisen DJ and Rosenberg S A: The in vivo distribution of autologous human and murine lymphoid cells grown in T cell growth factor (TCGF): Implications for the adoptive immunotherapy of tumors. J Immunol 1980 (125):1487-1493

5   Mazumder A, Grimm EA, Rosenberg SA: Lysis of fresh human solid tumor cells by autologous lymphocytes activated in vitro by allosensitization. Cancer Immunol Immunother 1983 (15):1-10

6   Rosenberg SA: Immunotherapy of cancer by the systemic administration of lymphoid cells plus interleukin-2. J Biol Resp Mod 1985 (3):501-511

7   Pizza G, Severini G, Menniti D et al: Tumour regression after intralesional injection of interleukin 2 (IL--2) in bladder cancer. Preliminary report. Int J Cancer 1984 (34):359-367

8   Lotze MT, Matory YL, Ettinghausen SE et al: In vivo administration of purified human interleukin 2. II. Half-life, immunologic effects, and expansion of peripheral lymphoid cells in vivo with recombinant IL-2. J Immunol 1985 (135):2865-2875

9   Atkins MB, Gould JA, Allegretta M et al: Phase I evaluation of recombinant interleukin-2 in patients with advanced malignant disease. Clin Oncol 1986 (4):1380-1391

10 Lotze MT, Chang AE, Seipp CA et al: High-dose recombinant interleukin 2 in the treatment of patients with disseminated cancer. JAMA 1986 (256):3117-3124

11 Lotze MT, Custer MC and Rosenberg SA: Intraperitoneal administration of interleukin-2 in patients with cancer. Arch Surg 1986 (121):1373-1379

12 Thompson JA, Lee DJ, Cox WW et al: Recombinant interleukin 2 toxicity, pharmacokinetics and immunomodulatory effects in a phase I trial. Cancer Res 1987 (47):4202-4207

13 Wang J, Walle A, Gordon B et al: Adoptive immunotherapy for stage IV renal cell carcinoma: a novel protocol utilizing periodate and interleukin 2 activated autologous leukocytes and continuous infusions of low dose interleukin 2. Am J Med 1987 (83):1016-1023

14 Yasumoto K, Miyazaki K, Nagashima A et al: Induction of lymphokine-activated killer cells by intrapleural instillations of recombinant interleukin-2 in patients with malignant pleurisy due to lung cancer. Cancer Res 1987 (47):2184-2187

15 Marolda R, Belli F, Prada A et al: A phase I study of recombinant interleukin 2 in melanoma patients. Toxicity and clinical effects. Tumori 1987 (73):575-584

16 Merguerian PA, Donahue L and Cockett ATK: Intraluminal interleukin 2 and Bacillus Calmette-Guerin for treatment of bladder cancer: A preliminary report. J Urol 1987 (137):216-219

17 Rosenberg SA: The development of new immunotherapies for the treatment of cancer using interleukin-2. Ann Surg 1988 (208):121-135

18 Sondel PM, Kohler PC, Hank JA et al: Clinical and immunological effects of recombinant interleukin 2 given by repetitive weekly cycles to patients with cancer. Cancer Res 1988 (48):2561-2567

19 Fisher RI, Coltman CA, Doroshow JH et al: Metastatic renal cancer treated with interleukin-2 and lymphokine activated killer cells. Ann Int Med 1988 (108):518-523

20 Thompson JA, Lee DJ, Lindgren CG et al: Influence of dose and duration of infusion of interleukin-2 on toxicity and immunomodulation. J Clin Oncol 1988 (6):669-678

21 Mitchell MS, Kempf RA, Harel W et al: Effectiveness and tolerability of low-dose cyclophosphamide and low-dose intravenous interleukin-2 disseminated melanoma. J Clin Oncol 1988 (6):409-424

22 Sosman JA, Kohler PC, Hank JA et al: Repetitive weekly cycles of interleukin-2. II. Clinical and immunologic effects of dose, schedule and additon of indomethacin. JNCI 1988 (80):1451-1461

23 Richards JM, Barker E, Latta J et al: Phase I study of weekly 24-hour infusions of recombinant human interleukin 2. JNCI 1988 (80):1325-1328

24 Pizza G, Viza D, De Vinci C et al: Intra-lymphatic administration of interleukin-2 (IL-2) in cancer patients: A pilot study. Lymphokine Res 1988 (7):45-48

25 Schoof DD, Gramolini BA, Davidson DL et al: Adoptive immunotherapy of human cancer using low-dose recombinant interleukin 2 and lymphokine-activated killer cells. Cancer Res 1988 (48):5007-5010

26 Krigel RL, Padavic-Shaller KA, Rudolph AR et al: A phase I study of recombinant interleukin 2 plus recombinant B-interferon. Cancer Res 1988 (48):3875-3881

27 Javadpour N and Lalehzarian M: A phase I-II study of high-dose recombinant human interleukin-2 in disseminated renal-cell carcinoma. Semin Surg Oncol 1988 (4):207-209

28 Yoshida S, Tanaka R, Takai N and Ono K: Local administration of autologous lymphokine-activated killer cells and recombinant interleukin 2 to patients with malignant brain tumours. Cancer Res 1988 (48):5011-5016

29 Cortesina G, De Stefani A, Giovarelli M et al: Treatment of recurrent squamous cell carcinoma of the head and neck with low doses of interleukin-2 injected perilymphatically. Cancer 1988 (62):2482-2485

30 Chapman PB, Kolitz JE, Hakes TB et al: A phase I trial of intraperitoneal recombinant interleukin 2 in

patients with ovarian carcinoma. Investig New Drugs 1988 (6):179-188

31 Merchant RE, Grant AJ, Merchant LH et al: Adoptive immunotherapy for recurrent glioblastoma multiforme using lymphokine activated killer cells and recombinant interleukin-2. Cancer 1988 (62):665-671

32 Onishi S, Saibara T, Fujikawa M et al: Adoptive immunotherapy with lymphokine-activated killer cells plus recombinant interleukin 2 in patients with unresectable hepatocellular carcinoma. Hepatology 1989 (10):349-353

33 Nasr S, McKolanis J, Pais R et al: A phase I study of interleukin-2 in children with cancer and evaluation of clinical and immunologic status during therapy. A Pediatric Oncology Group Study. Cancer 1989 (64):783-788

34 Stahel RA, Sculier JP, Jost LM et al: Tolerance and effectiveness of recombinant interleukin-2 (r-met Hu IL-2 [ala-125]) and lymphokine-activated killer cells in patients with metastatic solid tumors. Eur J Cancer Clin Oncol 1989 (25):965-972

35 Marumo K, Muraki J, Ueno M et al: Immunologic study of human recombinant interleukin-2 (low-dose) in patients with advanced renal cell carcinoma. Urology 1989 (33):219-225

36 Allison MAK, Jones SE and McGuffey P: Phase II trial of outpatient interleukin-2 in malignant lymphoma, chronic lymphocytic leukemia and selected solid tumors. J Clin Oncol 1989 (7):75-80

37 Paolozzi F, Zamkoff K, Doyle M et al: Phase I trial of recombinant interleukin-2 and recombinant B-interferon in refractory neoplastic disease. J Biol Resp Mod 1989 (8):122-139

38 Rosenberg SA, Lotze MT, Yang JC et al: Experience with the use of high-dose interleukin-2 in the treatment of 652 cancer patients. Ann Surg 1989 (210):474-442

39 Thatcher N, Dazzi H, Johnson RJ et al: Recombinant interleukin-2 (rIL-2) given intrasplenically and intravenously for advanced malignant melanoma. A phase I and II study. Br J Cancer 1989 (60):770-774

40 Sznol M, Dutcher JP, Atkins MB et al: Review of interleukin-2 alone and interleukin 2/ LAK clinical trials in metastatic malignant melanoma. Cancer Treat Rev 1989 (16 Suppl A):29-38

41 Stoter G, Shiloni E, Aamdal S et al: Sequential administration of recombinant human interleukin-2 and dacarbazine in metastatic melanoma. A multicentric phase II study. Eur J Cancer Clin Oncol 1989 (25 Suppl 3):S41-S43

42 Flaherty L: The combination of recombinant interleukin-2 and dacarbazine (DTIC) in metastatic malignant melanoma. Cancer Treat Rev 1989 (16 Suppl A):65-66

43 Lindermann A, Hoeffken K, Schmidt et al: A multicenter trial of interleukin-2 and low-dose cyclophosphamide in highly chemotherapy-resistant malignancies. Cancer Treat Rev 1989 (16 Suppl A):53-57

44 Paciucci PA, Holland JF, Ryder JS et al: Immunotherapy with interleukin-2 by constant infusion with and without adoptive cell transfer and with weekly doxorubicin. Cancer Treat Rev 1989 (16 Suppl A):67-81

45 West WH: Continuous infusion recombinant interleukin-2 (rIL-2) in adoptive cellular therapy of renal carcinoma and other malignancies. Cancer Treat Rev 1989 (16 Suppl A):83-89

46 Negrier S, Philip T, Stoter et al: Interleukin-2 with and without LAK cells in metastatic renal cell carcinoma: A report of a European multicentre study. Eur J Cancer Clin Oncol 1989 (25 Suppl 3):S21-S28

47 Panici PB, Scambia G, Greggi S et al: Recombinant interleukin-2 continuous infusion in ovarian cancer patients with minimal residual disease at second-look. Cancer Treat Rev 1989 (16 Suppl. A):123-127

48 Rosenberg SA, Lotze MT, Yang JC et al: Combination therapy with interleukin-2 and alpha-interferon for the treatment of patients with advanced cancer. J Clin Oncol 1989 (7):1863-1874

49 Lee KH, Talpaz M, Rothbeg JM et al: Concomitant administration of recombinant human interleukin-2 and recombinant alpha-2A in cancer patients: A phase I Study. J Clin Oncol 1989 (7):1726-1732

50 Thatcher N, Dazzi H, Mellor M et al: Recombinant interleukin-2 (rIL-2) with flavone acetic acid (FAA) in advanced malignant melanoma: a phase II study. Br J Cancer 1990 (61):618-621

51 Bukowski RM, Goodman P, Crawford ED et al: Phase II trial of high-dose intermittent interleukin-2 in metastatic renal cell carcinoma: A Southwest Oncology Group study. JNCI 1990 (82):143-146

52 Sondel PM, Hank JA, Kohler PC et al: The cellular immunotherapy of cancer: current and potential uses of interleukin-2. Crit Rev Oncol/Haematol 1989 (9):125-147

53 Sarna GP, Figlin RA, Pertcheck, M et al: Systemic administration of recombinant methionyl human interleukin-2 (Ala 125) to cancer patients: clinical results. J Biol Res Mod 1989 (8):16-24

54 Allegretta M, Atkins MB, Dempsey RA et al: The development of anti-interleukin-2 antibodies in patients treated with recombinant human interleukin-2 (IL-2). J Clin Immunol 1986 (6):481-489

55 Sano T, Saijo N, Sasaki Y et al: Three schedules of recombinant human interleukin-2 in the treatment of malignancy: side effects and immunologic effects in relation to serum level. Jpn J Cancer Res 1988 (79):131-143

56 Hank JA, Kohler PC, Weil-Hillman G et al: In vivo induction of the lymphokine-activated killer phenomenon: Interleukin-2 - dependent human non-major histocompatibility complex-restricted cytotoxicity generated in vivo during administration of human recombinant interleukin-2. Cancer Res 1988 (48):1965-1971

57 Creekmore P, Harris JE, Ellis TM et al: A Phase I clinical trial of recombinant interleukin-2 by periodic 24 hour intravenous infusions. J Clin Oncol 1989 (7):276-284

58 Ghosh AK, Dazzi H, Thatcher N and Moor M: Lack of correlation between peripheral blood lymphokine-activated killer (LAK) cell function and clinical response in patients with advanced malignant melanoma receiving recombinant interleukin 2. Int J Cancer (43):410-414

59 McMannis JD, Fisher RI, Creekmore SP et al: In vivo effects of Recombinant IL-2. I. Isolation of circulating Leu-19+ Lymphokine-Activated Killer effector cells from cancer patients receiving recombinant IL-2. J Immunology 1988 (140):1335-1340

60 Gambacorti-Passerini C, Rivoltini L, Radrizzani M et al: Differences between *in vivo* and *in vitro* activation of cancer patient lymphocytes by recombinant interleukin 2: Possible role for Lymphokine-Activated Killer cell infusion in the *in vitro* - induced activation. Cancer Res 1989 (49):5230-5234

61 Walewski J, Paietta E, Dutcher J and Wiernik PH: Evaluation of natural killer and lymphokine-activated killer (LAK) cell activity in vivo in patients treated with high-dose interleukin-2 and adoptive transfer of autologous LAK cells. J Cancer Res Clin Oncol 1989 (115):170-174

62 Boldt DH, Mills BJ, Gemlo BT et al: Laboratory correlates of adoptive immunotherapy with recombinant interleukin-2 and lymphokine-activated killer cells in humans. Cancer Res 1988 (48):4409-4416

63 Thompson JA, Lee DJ, Lindgren CG, et al: Influence of schedule of interleukin 2 administration on therapy with interleukin 2 and lymphokine activated killer cells. Cancer Res 1989 (49):235-240

64 Phillips J H and Lanier LL et al: Dissection of the lymphokine-activated killer phenomenon. Relative contribution of peripheral blood natural killer cells and T lymphocytes to cytolosis. J Exp Med 1986 (164):814-825

65 Gemlo BT, Palladino MA, Jaffe HS et al: Circulating cytokines in patients with metastatic cancer treated with recombinant interleukin 2 and lymphokine-activated killer cells. Cancer Res 1988 (48):5864-5867

66 Heslop HE, Gottlieb DJ, Bianchi AC et al: In vivo induction of gamma interferon and tumour necrosis factor by interleukin-2 infusion following intensive chemotherapy or autologous transplantation. Blood 1989 (4):1374-1380

67 Parkinson D: Interleukin-2 in cancer therapy. Semin Oncol 1988 (6 Suppl 6):10-26

68 De Fries RU and Golub SH: Characteristics and mechanism of IFN-induced protection of human tumour cells from lysis by lymphokine-activated killer cells. J Immunol 1988 (10):3686-3693

69 Lee RE, Lotze MT, Skibber JM et al: Cardiorespiratory effects of immunotherapy with interleukin-2. J Clin Oncol 1989 (7):7-20

70 Cotran RS, Pober JS, Gimbrone MA et al: Endothelial activation during interleukin 2 immunotherapy. A possible mechanism for the vascular leak syndrome. J Immunol 1987 (139):1883-1888

71 Mier JW, Brandon EP, Libby P et al: Activated endothelial cells resist lymphokine-activated killer cell-mediated injury. Possible role of induced cytokines in limiting capilliary leak during IL-2 therapy. J Immunol 1989 (143):2407-2414

72 Krigel RL, Padavic-Shaller KA, Rudolph AR et al: Exacerbation of epidemic Kaposi's sarcoma with a combination of interleukin-2 and beta-interferon: Results of a phase 2 study. J Biol Response Mod 1989 (8):359-365

73 Hamblin TJ: Interleukin-2. Side effects are acceptable. Br Med J 1990 (300):275-276

74 Herberman RB: Interleukin-2 therapy of human cancer: Potential benefits versus toxicity. J Clin Oncol 1989 (7):1-4

75 Eberlein TJ, Schoof DD, Michie HR et al: Ibuprofen causes reduced toxic effects of Interleukin 2 administration in patients with metastatic cancer. Arch Surg 1989 (124):542-547

76 Vetto JT, Papa MZ, Lotze MT et al: Reduction of toxicity of interleukin-2 and Lymphokine-Activated Killer cells in humans by the administration of corticosteroids J Clin Oncol 1987 (5):496-503

77 Belldegrun A, Webb D E, Austin HA et al: Renal toxicity of interleukin-2 administration in patients with metastatic renal cell cancer: Effect of pre-therapy nephrectomy. Urology 1989 (141):499-503

78 Javadpour N and Lalehzarian M: Role of interleukin 2 alone in disseminated renal cell carcinoma: An update. Prog Clin Biol Res 1989 (303) 671-679

79 Cohen PJ, Lotze MT, Roberts JR et al: The immunopathology of sequential tumour biopsies in patients treated with interleukin-2: Correlation of response with T-cell infiltration and HLA-DR expression. Am J Pathology 1987 (129):208-216

80 Atkins MB, Mier JW, Parkinson DR et al: Hypothyroidism after treatment with interleukin-2 and Lymphokine-Activated Killer cells. N Engl J Med 1988 (314):1557-1563

81 Kohler PC, Hank JA, Moore KH et al: Phase I clinical trial of recombinant interleukin-2: A comparison of bolus and continuous intravenous infusion. Cancer Investig 1989 (7):213-223

82 Kolitz JE, Welte K, Wong GY et al: Expansion of activated T-Lymphocytes in patients treated with recombinant interleukin 2. J Biol Resp Mod 1987 (6):412-429

83 Kay NE, Oken MM, Mazza JJ, Bradley EC: Evidence for tumor reduction in refractory or relapsed B-CLL patients with infusional interleukin 2. Nouv Rev Fr Hematol 1988 (30):475-478

84 Roth AD and Kirkwood JM: New clinical trials with interleukin-2: rationale for regional administration. Nat Immun Cell Growth Regul 1989 (8):153-164

85 Pizza G, Berton F, Casanova S et al: Interleukin 2 in the treatment of infiltrating bladder cancer. J Exp Path 1987 (3):525-531

86 Huland E and Huland H: Local continuous high dose interleukin 2: A new therapeutic model for the treatment of advanced bladder carcinoma. Cancer Res 1989 (49):5469-5474

87 Thatcher N, Taylor P, Carroll KB et al: Interleukin 2 in malignant pleural mesothelioma (and adenocarcinoma of the lung). The use of intrapleural and continuous intravenous infusions: preliminary results. Cancer Treat Rev 1989 (16 Suppl A):161-162

88 Kolitz JE, Wong GY, Welte K et al: Phase I trial of recombinant Interleukin 2 and cyclophosphamide: augmentation of cellular immunity and T-cell mitogenic response with long-term administration of rIL-2. J Biol Resp Mod 1988 (7):457-472

89 Stoter G, Shiloni E, Aamdal S et al: Sequential administration of recombinant human interleukin-2 and dacarbazine in metastatic melanoma. A multicentre phase II study. Eur J Cancer Clin Oncol 1989 (25 Suppl 3):S41-S43

90 Shiloni E, Pouillart P, Janssens J et al: Sequential dacarbazine chemotherapy followed by recombinant interleukin 2 in metastatic melanoma. A pilot multicentre phase I-II study. Eur J Cancer Clin Oncol 1989 (25 Suppl 3):S45-S49

91 Wagstaff J, Vermorken JB, Schwartsmann G et al: A progress report of a phase I study of Interferon gamma and interleukin 2 and some comments on the mechanism of the toxicity due to Interleukin 2. Cancer Treat Rev 1989 (16 Suppl A):105-109

Interleukin 2 and LAK Cells

Federico Calabresi and Enzo Maria Ruggeri

Department of Medical Oncology, Regina Elena National Cancer Institute, viale Regina Elena 291, 00161 Rome, Italy

Recent advances in cellular immunology, combined with extraordinary progress in biotechnology, has led to the development of new immunotherapeutic approaches to cancer treatment. One of these is adoptive immunotherapy, defined as the transfer of active cells with antitumour activity to a tumour-bearing host, in order to mediate a therapeutic effect [1-2].

Interleukin 2 (IL2), initially called the "T-Cell Growth Factor" [3], is a 15,000 dalton glycoprotein, produced by the helper lymphocytic subpopulation under the stimulus of mitogens or of a specific antigen. IL2 maintains the growth of the T-lymphoid cells in culture for a long time and mediates a wide variety of immuno-regulatory effects both *in vitro* and *in vivo*. *In vitro*, IL2 acts as a helper in type B and C immune responses increasing cytotoxic B-lymphocyte generation. IL2 may also mediate the immune function recovery of lymphocytes in an immunodeficiency state. *In vivo*, it increases NK activity and responsiveness to alloantigens [4].

The ability to generate and maintain antigen-specific T-cell clones has led to the identification of a T-cell receptor (IL2R). IL2R has two distinct polypeptide chains: alpha or p 75 (low affinity) and beta or p 55 (high affinity) identified by the anti-TAC antigen, each containing an IL2-binding site. High-affinity binding is believed to occur when IL2 interacts simultaneously with residues on both chains [5,6].

Recent reports by Kumar et al. suggest that the low-affinity IL2R plays an important role in the control of T-cell proliferation by providing a negative feed-back influence [7]. These authors showed that:

a) high-affinity IL2R and IL2 complexes are internalised, while low-affinity IL2R and IL2 complexes are not;
b) following cell activation, the ratio of low- to high-affinity IL2Rs increases;
c) cell restimulation with IL2 provides a minor proliferative response when this ratio is higher.

At low concentrations, some monoclonal antibodies raised against IL2Rs cause a down-regulation of the low affinity IL2Rs, stimulating rather than suppressing cell proliferation.

Cytotoxic cell generation, *in vitro* and *in vivo*, depends on the presence of both IL2 and IL2R on the cell surface. Methods to increase IL2R expression could, therefore, be important to maximise cytotoxic cell proliferation. In this regard, gamma-interferon induces IL2R expression on peripheral blood T-lymphocytes [8-10].

When IL2 acts on peripheral blood lymphocytes, it induces gamma-interferon production leading to a positive feedback loop. Gamma-interferon, in turn, enhances the receptor expression and magnifies the helper effects of IL2 with its further production. Simultaneously, lymphocytes are committed to cell-cycle progression when stimulated by IL2 [10,11]. These studies provide the rationale for clinical studies on the IL2 + gamma-interferon combination.

IL2 receptors cannot be detected on most freshly isolated T-cells and appear asynchronously after the polyclonal activation of T-cell receptors. Within 3 days of activation, all cells express IL2 receptors. Thereafter, the receptor levels decline, perhaps as a result of a down-regulation by secreted IL2. Proliferation then ceases and the cells go into the cell cycle resting phase [12].

Lymphokine-Activated Killer (LAK) Cells

Rosenberg et al. first described a technique for generating lymphoid cells from both mice and humans. The incubation of resting murine splenocytes or human peripheral blood lymphocytes with IL2 occurs 3 to 4 days later in cell generation [13,14]. These cells are called lymphokine-activated killer (LAK) cells [15,16].

The term "LAK cell activity" describes the *in vitro* lysis of both autologous and allogeneic fresh tumour cells together with cultured tumour cell lines, including those resistant to lysis by NK cells. The LAK cell population is a heterogeneous lytic population, distinct from NK cells and cytolytic T-lymphocytes. Their phenotypic surface markers are characteristic of non-MHC restricted killer cells. Moreover, most of the cells mediating LAK activity are lymphocytes which belong to the null cell population. These were found to be predominantly Leu-11+ and are a strong source of NK activity [17-19].

At the present time, the biology of these different cell populations, their target specificities and response to various cytokines are unknown.

The adoptive administration of LAK cells + IL2 may elicit antitumour effects in the host. In experimental animal models, a regression of pulmonary and hepatic metastases of various tumours has been observed with IL2 alone and, to a much greater extent, with IL2 + LAK cells. The IL2 + LAK cell combination resulted in a significant reduction of liver metastases as compared to IL2 alone, showing a dose-effect relationship [20,21]. These observations have provided the rationale for the use of adoptive immunotherapy for metastatic human cancer.

Clinical Studies

Various studies have shown that different doses and schedules of IL2 elicit definite antineoplastic activity. The administration modality influences the response. Intravenous bolus administration rapidly produces high concentrations followed by a rapid fall, while administration by continuous infusion induces a greater IL2 concentration in the serum and target organs for a longer period of time.

Rosenberg et al. first reported the promising results obtained with the IL2 + LAK cells combination and with IL2 alone [22]. In the last update of this non-randomised study on 222 patients (139 treated with IL2 + LAK cells and 83 only with high-dose IL2), the following results were obtained: 12 complete responses (CRs) and 17 partial responses (PRs) in the IL2 + LAK cells group and 4 CRs and 9 PRs in the group treated only with IL2 [23]. The schedule is shown in detail in Figure 1.

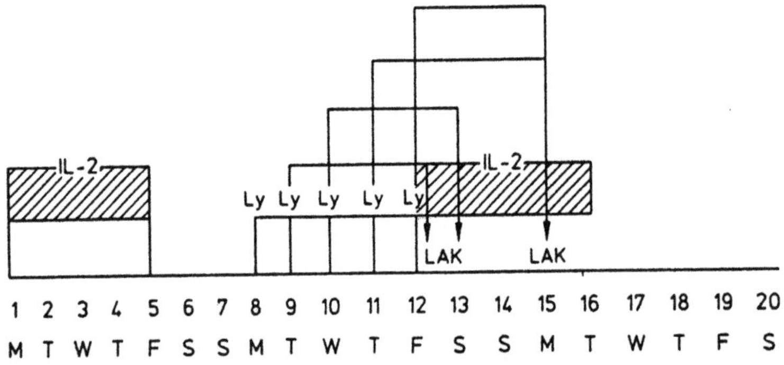

Fig.1. Rosenberg's first administration schedule of IL2 + LAK
Ly = Lymphocytapheresis; IL2 = 100,000 U/Kg iv q 8 hours
LAK = LAK cell infusion

Table 1. Response duration (months)

| Diagnosis | LAK + IL 2 | | IL 2 | |
	CR	PR	CR	PR
Renal cell carcinoma	14+, 12+, 9+, 9 7+, 6, 2+	15+, 11+, 6+, 6 6, 6, 6, 2, 1, 1	13+, 7+, 6+ 4+	7+, 7, 3
Melanoma	31+, 11+, 11+	6, 2, 2,	- 8, 7, 2	20, 12+, 10
Non-Hodgkin's lymphoma	10	11+, 7+	-	-
Colorectal carcinoma	17+	6, 2	-	-

source [23]

Regression of metastatic cancer was observed in patients with malignant melanoma, renal cell and colorectal carcinoma and non-Hodgkin's lymphoma. The primary sites of response included the lung, liver, bone, skin and subcutaneous tissue.

It is too early to establish the median CR duration for the entire group (range, 2 - 31+ months); the median duration of the PRs was 6 months (Table 1). A randomised trial comparing these two treatment modalities is currently in progress at the National Cancer Institute (NCI).

In another non-randomised phase II trial of the NCI Extramural Working Group, the IL2 + LAK cells combination was tested in 35 renal cell cancer patients [24]. An overall 16% response rate was obtained, 2 patients presenting a CR and 3 a PR. The complete responders were disease free at 9 and 12 months, while the PRs were maintained for 4, 15 and 16 months, showing results similar to those reported by Rosenberg.

To preserve the efficacy and reduce the toxicity of this treatment, West et al. employed escalating doses of IL2, administered as a constant infusion rather than in bolus [25]. In the first published report on 40 evaluable patients, 13 showed a PR and 2 a minor response. All the responses occurred in patients treated with the higher IL2 dose. The time to maximum response ranged from 15 to 30 days and the response duration from 1.5 to >7 months. The main response sites included the lymph nodes, lung, skin and soft

tissue. Toxicity was milder than that observed with the bolus IL2 administration, thanks to a simple interruption or reduction of the IL2 infusion until the toxic effects were resolved.

Sosman and Sondel demonstrated that low IL2 doses, given at prolonged administration schedules, provide acceptable toxicity rates and can induce an objective antitumour response (3 PRs in 23 renal cell carcinoma patients) [26-27]. Moreover, a marked increase in the number of activated, IL2-dependent circulating lymphocytes was observed together with a >100-fold increase in the cytotoxic potential of the expanded systemic lymphoid mass cells.

Thompson et al. analysed various IL2 dose levels (300,000 U/m^2/day and 3 MU/m^2/day), administered by 2- and 24-hour infusions [28]. The same high IL2 dose (3 MU/m^2/day) administered by i.v. bolus 3 times a day was also studied. All the doses were administered 5 days a week for 4 weeks. At equivalent total daily doses, the continuous IL2 infusion was more toxic and more biologically active with regard to post-IL2 lymphocytosis, circulating activated lymphocyte generation and LAK cell precursors. The greater toxicity of this administration contrasts with that reported by West and other authors, employing lower daily doses [25,29,30].

Paciucci et al. treated 25 disseminated cancer patients by continuous IL2 infusion and adoptive transfer of activated cells [31]. Infusions were given 6 days a week for 4 consecutive weeks, immediately following

Table 2. Results obtained with IL 2 + LAK cell immunotherapy (collected series)

| | IL 2 + LAK | | IL 2 alone | |
Tumour	No. pts.	OR	No. pts.	OR
Kidney	134	35	55	10
Melanoma	72	20	41	8
Colorectum	49	4	31	0
Non-Hodgkin's lymphoma	14	5		
Sarcoma	10	1		

OR = overall response (complete + partial)

transfusion of activated autologous lymphocytes. The IL2 dose was escalated weekly in each patient and in subsequent cohorts of patients until a maximum tolerated dose was reached. Objective tumour regression was noted in 9 patients (6 PRs, 2 minor responses and 1 mixed response). The responses were related to the IL2 dose and to the *in vivo* lymphoproliferative effects of the lymphokine but not to the number of adoptively transfused cells. The median response duration was 16 weeks (range, 3 - 60+ weeks).

These findings suggest that non-specific IL2 immunotherapy may be best employed in a minimal disease setting or as adjuvant treatment following surgical, radiotherapeutic or chemotherapeutic debulking.

In a phase I trial, Creekmore et al. investigated the immunomodulation and toxicity of 24-hour continuous IL2 infusion [32]. Thirty-three patients were treated with weekly or twice weekly 24-hour infusions. Two PRs, one minor response and one mixed response were obtained in patients with soft tissue, adrenal and liver metastases.

Interesting findings were obtained with regard to immunomodulatory effects. As the IL2 dosage increased, so did the immunomodulation. All patients who received one or more doses of IL2 at 3 MU/m^2/day (the maximum tolerated dose) developed LAK effector cells in the peripheral blood. The most striking finding, however, was the generation of large numbers of circulating Leu 19+ cells with a tolerable toxicity for patients treated twice weekly at this dosage. In these patients, the number of Leu 19+ cells is comparable to that infused with *ex vivo* generated LAK cell treatment, as in the Rosenberg protocol. However, the endogenously generated Leu 19+ cells may not be identical to laboratory-generated LAK cells.

To reduce the side effects of IL2, Mitchell et al. treated 24 melanoma patients with IL2 + cyclophosphamide (350 mg/m^2) [33]. Objective responses were observed in 25% of the patients (1 CR and 5 PRs). The main sites of response were the liver, the lymph nodes and the lungs. This study indicated that this combination may be useful in reducing toxicity and improving therapeutic efficacy.

A collected series of tumour type responses is summarised in Table 2 [23-28,31-35].

Eberlein et al. employed low-dose systemic IL2 (over a prolonged administration period) and LAK cells [34]. No hypotension requiring vasopressors, pulmonary oedema nor changes in mental state were observed. When employing Ibuprofen (600 mg p.o. every 6 hours), these authors observed a reduction of minor side effects (fever, chills, nausea and vomiting). In 40 consecutive patients treated, 4 CRs and 12 PRs were observed, showing an overall response rate of 40%. Responses were obtained in 5 out of 12 renal carcinomas, 8 out of 16 melanomas, 2 out of 4 lymphomas and 1 out of 2 ovarian carcinomas. The responses lasted from 1 to 19+ months.

Thompson et al. treated 12 patients (4 with melanoma and 8 with renal cell carcinoma) with a continuous high-dose IL2 infusion (6 MU/m^2/day) and LAK cells. Significant toxicity was observed in 6 patients, requiring intensive-care hospitalisation. No melanoma patients responded and 1 CR and 2 PRs were observed in patients with a higher LAK-cell yield [35].

Table 3. Patient characteristics

Sex: Male = 13   Female = 12

Median age: 50.5 years (range, 24-68 years)

Median ECOG performance status: 1 (range, 0-2)

Diagnosis		**Prior therapy**	
Melanoma	14	S + CT + IT	7
Renal cell carcinoma	7	S	4
Hodgkin's lymphoma	2	S + CT	3
Colorectal carcinoma	1	S + IT	2
Adrenal carcinoma	1	S + CT + HT	2
		S + RT	1
No. of metastatic sites		RT + CT	1
1 site = 10 patients		RT + CT + IT	1
2 sites = 11 patients		RT + CT + BMT	1
3 or more sites = 4 patients		S + IT + HT + CT	1

S = surgery; CT = chemotherapy; IT = immunotherapy; HT = hyperthermia; RT = radiotherapy; BMT = bone marrow transplantation

The administration schedule of IL2 (bolus or continuous infusion) remains controversial. In a randomised phase II study, Weiss et al. treated 61 renal cell carcinoma patients with LAK cells and IL2 by bolus injection or continuous infusion [36]. No significant differences between the two treatment modalities were observed with regard to efficacy, toxicity or LAK activation.

In 1987, a phase I-II trial with IL2 + LAK was initiated at the Regina Elena National Cancer Institute in collaboration with the Laboratory of Haematology of the University of Rome and the Laboratory of Haematology and Oncology of the Italian National Institute of Health [37]. The trial was conducted on patients with metastatic disease who had not responded to conventional therapy, according to Rosenberg's original protocol.

To date, a total of 25 patients have been treated, 13 males and 12 females (Table 3). The median age was 50.5 years (range, 24-68 years; performance status, 0 to 1 in 24 patients and 2 in 1 patient). There were 14 patients with melanoma, 7 with renal cell carcinoma, 2 with Hodgkin's disease, 1 with adrenal carcinoma and 1 with colorectal carcinoma. Escalating doses of IL2 (Hoffman-La Roche, provided by the NCI) were administered to 4 groups of patients. The first 3 groups were composed of 5 patients each receiving 1 MU/m^2, 3 MU/m^2 and 4.5 MU/m^2 3 times a day. The fourth group, which received 6 MU/m^2/x3/day, was extended to 10 patients because of the severe toxicity observed in the first 5, to establish if this is the maximum tolerated dose. The total quantities of IL2 and LAK cells administered are shown in Table 4.

Table 4. Total IL 2 and LAK cells administered

Group	No. pts.	IL 2 (x 10^6)		LAK cells (x 10^9)	
		Median	Range	Median	Range
I	5	52	31.5 - 54	20.1	9.1 - 45
II	5	144	93 - 156	30	16.5 - 40.3
III	5	154	129 - 175	20	18.5 - 46.6
IV	10	235	150 - 230	39.5	4.6 - 75.4

Table 5.   Treatment response

Group	No.pts.	PR	SD	P	Duration (months)
I	5	-	2	3	4 - 24+
II	5	-	2	3	3 - 9
III	5	2	-	3	4 - 12.5+
IV	10	-	1	9	3+

Two patients presented a PR of 4 and 12.5+ months' duration, 5 presented stable disease of 3, 5, 9 and 24+ months' duration and 18 patients showed progressive disease. The two PRs were obtained in melanoma patients both pertaining to the third group (Table 5). LAK cells monitored by immunoscintigraphy did not show any selective homing to tumour sites. The toxicity observed may be considered acceptable. Oliguria, hypotension, thrombocytopenia and weight gain were dose related while cutaneous and hepatic toxicity, fever and diarrhoea were constantly present, regardless of the dose. The symptoms, however, were reversible shortly after suspension of the therapy.

Our limited experience appears to confirm the activity of adoptive immunotherapy for patients with melanoma. For future phase II studies employing this same regimen, a dosage of 4.5 MU/m^2 is recommended.

Toxicity and Supportive Care

As most studies point to a strong dose-response relationship, the major goal of clinical trials has been to administer the maximum tolerated dose of IL2 with an acceptable toxicity level. Unfortunately, however, the high IL2 dosages required for LAK production often cause severe toxicity, sometimes requiring intensive-care hospitalisation.

While the morbidity rate of this treatment is high, the mortality rate (2%) is comparable to that observed employing standard chemotherapeutic regimens.

The principal side effect of IL2 administration is an increased vascular permeability, the "capillary leak syndrome", probably due to the release of histamine-like substances such as prostaglandins, or to the direct effects of the cytokines on the endothelium [38-41].

Nearly all patients experience hypotension, which may be treated initially with fluids. However, most patients have an increase in body weight of up to 10% and develop oedema or pleural effusion. Colloid solutions and vasopressor agents are administered when fluids are contraindicated (i.e., in the presence of the capillary leak syndrome).

Oliguria may be considered a direct effect of the increased vascular permeability due to the passage of fluids into the extravasal space. Hypotension obviously worsens this effect and diuretics are often not helpful. IL2-induced changes in renal tubular functions, suggesting a specific damage, have also been observed.

All patients show high azotemia and serum creatinine levels. Baseline serum creatinine values of more than 1.5 mg/dl are associated with greater renal toxicity [42].

Myocardial toxicity during the course of IL2 treatment was first reported by Rosenberg [2]. Supraventricular tachycardia, atrial fibrillation, premature supraventricular and ventricular beating, and myocardial infarction have also been reported. At the present time, it is not certain whether the myocardial infarction is a result of the capillary leak syndrome in patients with an underlying coronary artery disease or whether IL2 directly or indirectly damages the cardiac muscle. A reduction of the left ventricular ejection fraction, however, was always observed [38].

Pleural effusion caused by the "capillary leak syndrome" is frequently found at various IL2 dosages, while dispnoea, requiring intubation, may be present at higher dosages.

During leukapheresis, anaemia is common and blood trasfusions are required. Thrombocytopenia may develop during treatment but no haemorrhagic complications have ever been reported.

Confusion, drowsiness and disorientation have also been described, so that any change in mental state should be carefully examined. Neuropsychiatric side effects require more recovery time after treatment interruption.

Hepatic enzyme abnormalities are often observed. High transaminase, bilirubin and al-

Table 6. IL 2 toxicity and treatment

Toxicity	Symptom	Therapy
Systemic	Chills	Antihistamines Meperidine
	Fever	Acetaminophen-Indomethacin
Cardiopulmonary	Arrhythmia	Digoxin Verapamil
	Hypotension	Fluids-colloids Vasopressors
	Dyspnoea	Oxygen Bicarbonate
	Pleural effusion	Thoracentesis (if indicated)
Renal	Oliguria	Fluids-diuretics Vasopressors
Gastrointestinal	Nausea and vomiting	Metoclopramide
	Diarrhoea	Loperamide Dyphenoxilate hydrochloride
Haematological	Anaemia	Blood transfusions
Dermatological	Dry desquamation	Oil liniment
	Pruritus	Hydroxyzine hydrochloride
Neuropsychiatric	Hallucinations	Witheld IL 2
	Stupor and coma	Steroids
Infective		Antibiotics

kaline phosphatase levels are not always dose related.

Nausea and vomiting may be controlled by antiemetic drugs. Diarrhoea can be severe and may sometimes cause hypokalaemia or acidosis. Patients can also experience chills requiring antihistamines and, if these are insufficient, meperidine. To prevent or cure fever, acetaminophen and indomethacin are employed.

Extended rashes, pruritus and skin desquamation are frequent, while stomatitis and glossitis are never severe and require only local medication. In addition, all patients experience anorexia, flu-like syndrome and arthralgia.

However, all of these side effects are reversible and resolve within 24 to 48 hours after interrupting therapy.

The endocrine effects of IL2 are particularly interesting and consist of two general types: either as a consequence of an acute inflammatory response induction or as more chronic changes associated with an autoimmune disease. The adrenocorticotrophic hormone, cortisol, prolactin and growth hormone levels have all been discovered to rise after IL2 treatment.

Atkins et al. recently demonstrated hypothyroidism development in 20% of the patients treated, although those developing this deficiency presented preexisting thyroid autoantibodies [44]. Decreasing thyroxine levels combined with increasing thyroid-stimulating hormone levels were noted, sometimes together with marked hypothyroidism. The fact that the objective response rate was much higher in patients who developed hypothyroidism than in those who remained euthyroid is interesting. Conventional thyroid substitute therapy can control this effect.

Biological Effects

Most of the biological effects observed during IL2 treatment are mediated by the secretion of other lymphokines or cytokines possessing *in vitro* antitumour activity. The highest serum cytokine levels (IFN-gamma, TNF-alpha, TNF-beta) occur following LAK-cell infusion [45]. The cytokine response to LAK-cell infusion varies depending on the treatment schedule. Patients receiving bolus IL2 during cell reinfusion more frequently develop higher cytokine levels than those receiving the continuous infusion. These differences, however, do not appear to be related to the number of LAK cells reinfused.

In the study we conducted on patients receiving IL2 + LAK cell treatment, serum levels of soluble IL2R (sIL2R), B2-microglobulin (B2-M), a non-glycosylated protein which forms the light chain of the class I MHC, and IFN were studied [46]. The following results were found:

a) A significant sIL2R increase with peak levels on day 3 or 4. (Parallel immunofluorescence studies showed that the percentage of IL2R peripheral blood lymphocytes significantly increased during IL2 immunotherapy and that IL2 induces preferentially low-affinity sIL2R.)

b) Following IL2 administration, serum B2-M concentrations increase significantly.

c) Gamma-IFN levels increase at an early stage during IL2 therapy, reaching peak levels on day 1 or 2 with considerable differences between one patient and the other.

Wiebke et al. evaluated cell-mediated immunity, measured by delayed-type hypersensitivity skin testing in patients submitted to adoptive immunotherapy with IL2 + LAK cells. In particular, the effects of IL2 and LAK cells on acute delayed-type hypersensitivity responses were studied [47]. Nine out of 10 patients developed anergy during therapy. This drop was higher after LAK cell reinfusion as compared to pretreatment (p < 0.01) and post IL2 alone (p = 0.04).

It should be specified that skin testing is representative of the global immune status of the host and not just of specific T-lymphocytes mediating a delayed-type hypersensitivity.

In fact, flow cytometry revealed sharp increases in T-lymphocyte counts after IL2 alone and in IL2 receptor-bearing cells but not in the number of B-lymphocyte or monocyte counts.

Prognostic Factors

As we have seen, adoptive immunotherapy with LAK cells or IL2 can cause tumour regression in patients who do not respond to other available therapy. But which patients are most likely to respond?

West et al. report that the treatment response is related to the pretreatment performance status (0-1 vs. 2; p < 0.01) [25]. They also observed that the likelihood of a response is related to baseline lymphocyte counts ($1531/mm^3$ vs. $898/mm^3$; p < 0.01) and to the degree of lymphocytosis produced by the priming exposure to IL2 ($7997/mm^3$ vs. $3771/mm^3$; p < 0.01). These same authors report that mononuclear cells of responding patients have a slightly higher number of lytic units per 10^7 cells after *in vitro* activation, although these differences were not statistically significant.

Creekmore et al. found no differences in the levels of circulating effector cells between responders and non-responders [28].

Paciucci et al. examined the relationship between tumour regression and IL2 dose [31]. A correlation was found between higher IL2 doses and tumour regression (p = 0.44) but not between the number of activated transfused cells and tumour response. Rebound lymphocytosis following IL2 infusion correlates with antitumour effects (p = 0.008), while no correlation has been observed for eosinophils or total WBC counts.

Mitchell et al. found no correlation with tumour response when evaluating tumour burden, number of LAK cells administered, degree of toxicity induced, amount of IL2 administered or other treatment characteristics [33]. By examining the series of renal cell cancer patients reported by Rosenberg, together with their own patients from the IL2/LAK Extramural Working Group, Fisher et al. demonstrated that patients with pulmonary metastases or soft tissue disease are more likely to respond than patients with abdominal disease. Lower response rates were also observed in patients with a single tumour mass > 100 cm^2 and in patients who had not been submitted to prior nephrectomy [24].

There are evidently conflicting data regarding possible prognostic factors. No multivariate analysis is available because of the small number of patients entered into the various trials. Tumour type, extent of disease, pretreatment immunobiological status of the patients and other patient characteristics are all factors that may influence the outcome of these treatments.

Tumour-Infiltrating Lymphocytes

New immunotherapeutic approaches have led investigators to study more effective and less toxic protocols, employing different lymphoid cells. Experimental models on mice have identified tumour-infiltrating lymphocytes (TILs) that show high antineoplastic activity, both *in vivo* and *in vitro* [48].

TILs are a lymphoid subgroup present in the tumour mass which may be selectively expanded by digestive enzymatic processes of the tumour in the presence of IL2 [13]. They differ from LAK cells for the following reasons [48,49]:

1) high TIL doses may exert antineoplastic effects regardless of IL2 administration, although its effectiveness is increased at least 5-fold when combined with IL2;
2) in 95% of the cases, TILs cultured in IL2 are cytotoxic T-cells;
3) TILs have a greater lytic effect against fresh autologous tumour cells and show a lytic specificity for the autologous target;

4) pretreatment with a single dose of cyclophosphamide greatly increases the efficacy of transferred TILs. TILs can be extracted and expanded from various tumours when stimulated by mitogens or lymphokines [50-54].

In an immunotherapy trial employing human TILs, Kradin et al. showed that more than 10^9 autologous TILs could be transferred to patients with lung cancer [55]. Some showed a slight tumour response to treatment and increased delayed-type hypersensitivity responses to recall antigens.

Rosenberg et al. treated 20 patients with metastatic melanoma with the adoptive transfer of TILs and IL2 after therapy with a single cyclophosphamide dose [56]. An objective response was achieved in 9 out of 15 patients (60%) who had not been previously treated with IL2 and in 2 out of 5 (40%) in whom previous IL2 therapy failed. The response duration ranged from 2 to 13+ months. Moreover, the same group demonstrated that labelled TILs can localise preferentially at the tumour site as early as 24 hours after injection [57].

Kradin et al. observed an 18% response rate in 28 evaluable patients with malignant melanoma, renal cell carcinoma and non small-cell lung carcinoma [58]. Partial responses were obtained in 3 out of 13 melanoma patients and in 2 out of the 7 renal cell carcinoma patients.

Tumour reduction occurred within 4 to 12 weeks and lasted from 3 to 11 months. The toxic effects were correlated to the IL2 dose but no hypotension requiring vasopressors, anuria, or pulmonary oedema were observed.

These early results with TILs are encouraging but further investigations regarding this approach are required.

Conclusions

The observation that solid tumours can regress by modifying the patient's immune system opens an entirely new and more natural field of research.

Interleukin 2, alone or in combination with LAK cells, is therapeutically effective, especially in malignant melanoma and renal cell carcinoma. The rationale for employing IL2 has been to stimulate endogenous NK activity which can have a therapeutic activity against established metastases, expand the effector population *in vivo* and/or maintain the adoptively transferred LAK cell activity.

Since the role of LAK cells does not appear to be as significant in clinical practice as in experimental models, their nature and functions must be further explored. The procedures for leukapheresis should be improved and the cultured lymphocytes must be more specific in order to determine a selective homing to tumour sites. Only in this manner will it be possible to understand whether LAK cells are specific antitumour agents or simply an aspecific immunological reinforcement.

IL2 has been administered at various doses and schedules (in bolus or by continuous infusion) but no definite conclusions can be drawn regarding the superiority of one over the other. The toxicity related to IL2 treatment is the most serious problem to be resolved inasmuch as the mortality rate is low but the morbidity rate is high.

The following questions must still be answered:

1) Is toxicity a necessary counterpart of the beneficial effects?
2) How can the capillary leak syndrome be avoided?
3) Do steroids affect tumour response?
4) What is the role of indomethacin?
5) How can patients who are most likely to respond to adoptive immunotherapy be selected?

The lymphocyte count, the presence of lung metastases, the extension of the tumour mass and the number of adoptive transferred cells have all been considered [24,25,31,32].

New methods are currently being developed to enhance the immunotherapeutic efficacy of IL2. Some of these have already been included in ongoing clinical trials (TILs, TNFs and cytokine combinations) and represent a base for significant improvements in cancer treatment.

The possibility of transferring immunobiologically active cells to a tumour-bearing host opens an exciting new field of research. The experimental bases and the positive results obtained in animals have only partially been confirmed in human cancer. At present, there are many more questions than answers regarding adoptive immunotherapy. Only more extensive studies conducted on a larger number of patients will enable us to evaluate the true role of this new cancer treatment.

REFERENCES

1 Rosenberg SA: The adoptive immunotherapy of cancer. Accomplishments and prospects. Cancer Treat Rep 1984 (68):233-255

2 Rosenberg SA: Adoptive immunotherapy of cancer using lymphokine activated killer cells and recombinant interleukin-2. In: De Vita VT, Hellman S, Rosenberg SA (eds) Important Advances in Oncology. JB Lippincott, Philadelphia 1986, pp 55-91

3 Morgan DA, Ruscetti FW and Gallo RC: Selective in vitro growth of T Lymphocytes from normal human bone marrows. Science 1976 (193):1007-1008

4 Parkinson DR: Interleukin-2 in cancer therapy. Sem Oncol 1988 (15 suppl 6):10-26

5 Tsudo M, Kozak RW, Goldman CK et al: Demonstration of a non-TAC peptide that binds interleukin-2: a potential partecipant in a multichain interleukin-2 receptor complex. Proc Natl Acad Sci USA 1986 (83):9694-9698

6 Teshigawara K, Wang HM, Kato K et al: Interleukin-2 high affinity receptor expression requires to distinct binding protein. J Exp Med 1987 (165):225-238

7 Kumar A, Moreau JL, Beran D et al: Evidence for negative regulation of T cell growth by low affinity interleukin-2 receptors. J Immunol 1987 (138):1485

8 Kashara T, Hoors JJ, Dougherty ST et al: Interleukin-2 mediated immune interferon production by human T cells and T cell subsets. J Immunol 1983 (130):1784

9 Riccardic Vose BM and Herberman RB: Modification of IL-2 dependent growth of mouse NK cells by interferon and T lymphocytes. J Immunol 1983 (130):228

10 Johnson HM and Farran WL: The role of y-interferon like lymphokine in the activation of T cells for expression of interleukin receptors. Cell Immunol 1983 (75):154

11 Kurivayashi K, Gilles S, Kern DE et al: Murine cell cultures: effects of interleukin-2 and interferon on cell growth and cytotoxic reactivity. J Immunol Mol Biol 1984 (126):2321

12 Smith KA: Interleukin-2, inception, impact and implications. Lancet 1988 (240):1169-1176

13 Yron I, Wood TA, Spiess R and Rosenberg SA: In vitro growth of murine T cells: V. The isolation and growth of lymphoid cells infiltrating syngeneic solid tumors. J Immunol 1980 (125):238-245

14 Lotze MT, Grimm E, Mazumder A et al: In vitro growth of cytotoxic human lymphocytes: IV. Lysis of fresh and cultured autologous tumor by lymphocytes cultured in T cell growth factor (TCGF). Cancer Res 1981 (41):4420-4425

15 Grimm EA, Mazumder A, Zhang HZ and Rosenberg SA: The lymphokine activated killer cell phenomenon: lysis of NK resistant fresh solid tumor by IL-2 activated autologous human peripheral blood lymphocytes. J Exp Med 1982 (155):1823-1841

16 Rayner AA, Grimm EA, Lotze MT et al: Lymphokine activated killer (LAK) cell phenomenon. Analysis of factors relevant to the immunotherapy of human cancer. Cancer 1985 (55):1327-1333

17 Grimm EA, Ramsey KM, Mazumder A et al: Lymphokine-activated killer cells phenomenon: II. The precursor phenotype is serologically distinct from peripheral T-Lymphocytes, memory CTL and NK cells. J Exp Med 1983 (157):884-897

18 Rosenstein M, Yron I, Kaufmann Y and Rosenberg SA: Lymphokine-activated killer cells: Lysis of fresh syngeneic NK-resistant murine tumor cells by lymphocytes cultured in IL-2. Cancer Res 1984 (44):1946-1953

19 Roberts K, Lotze MT and Rosenberg SA: Separation and functional studies of the human lymphokine-activated killer cells. Cancer Res 1987 (47):4366-4371

20 Lafreniere R and Rosenberg SA: Successful immunotherapy of murine experimental hepatic metastases with lymphokine activated killer cells and recombinant Interleukin-2. Cancer Res 1985 (45):3735-3741

21 Mazumder A and Rosenberg SA: Successful immunotherapy of natural killer-resistant established pulmonary melanoma metastases by the intravenous adoptive transfer of syngeneic lymphocytes activated in vitro by Interleukin-2. J Exp Med 1984 (159):495-507

22 Rosenberg SA, Lotze MT, Munl LM et al: Observations on the systemic administration of autologous lymphokine-activated killer cells and recombinant Interleukin-2 to patients with metastatic cancer. N Engl J Med 1985 (313):1485-1492

23 Rosenberg SA: The development of new immunotherapies for the treatment of cancer using Interleukin-2. Am Surg 1988 (208):121-135

24 Fisher RI, Coltman CA Jr, Doroshaw JH et al: Metastatic renal cell cancer treated with Interleukin-2 and lymphokine-activated killer cells. Ann Intern Med 1988 (108):518-523

25 West WH, Taner KW, Yannelli JR et al: Constant-infusion recombinant Interleukin-2 in adoptive immunotherapy of advanced cancer. N Engl J Med 1987 (316):898-905

26 Sosman JA, Kohler PC, Hank J et al: Repetitive weekly cycles of recombinant human Interleukin-2: Responses of renal carcinoma with acceptable toxicity. JNCI 1988 (80):60-63

27 Sondel PM, Kohler PC and Hank JA: Clinical and immunological effects of recombinant Interleukin-2 given by repetitive weekly cycles to patients with cancer. Cancer Res 1988 (48):2561-2567

28 Thompson MS, Kempf RA, Harel W et al: Influence of dose and duration of infusion of Interleukin-2 on toxicity and immunomodulation. J Clin Oncol 1988 (4):668

29 Paciucci PA, Bhardwaj S, Odchimar R et al: Immunotherapy for metastatic cancer with recombinant Interleukin-2 (rIL-2) by continuous infusion with and without adoptive cell transfer. Proc Am Soc Clin Oncol 1988 (7):163

30 Richards JM, Vogelzang NJ, Ramming K et al: Preliminary results of a randomized trial of recombinant human Interleukin-2 (rIL-2) given by continuous venous infusion (CVI) with or without lymphokine activated killer cells (LAK). Proc Am Soc Clin Oncol 1988 (7):160

31 Paciucci PA, Holland JF, Glidewell O et al: Recombinant Interleukin-2 by continuous infusion and adoptive transfer of recombinant Interleukin-2 activated cells in patients with advanced cancer. J Clin Oncol 1989 (7):869-878

32 Creekmore SP, Harris JE, Ellis JM et al: A phase I clinical trial of recombinant Interleukin-2 by periodic 24 hours Intravenous Infusion. J Clin Oncol 1989 (7):276-284

33 Mitchell MS, Kempf RA, Harel W et al: Effectiveness and tolerability of low dose cyclophosphamide and low dose interleukin-2 in disseminated melanoma. J Clin Oncol 1988 (3):401-424

34 Eberlein TS, Lorenz K, Martell K et al: Low dose recombinant Interleukin-2 (rIL-2) and lymphokine-activated killer (LAK) cells - reduced toxicity: An alternative to high-dose rIL-2/high toxicity. Prot Soc Am Clin Oncol 1989 (8):180

35 Thompson J, Lee D, Benz L et al: High-dose continuous intravenous (CIV) infusion Interleukin-2 (IL-2) and lymphokine-activated killer (LAK) cell therapy for renal cell carcinoma and melanoma. Proc Soc Am Clin Oncol 1989 (8):181

36 Weiss GR, Margolin K, Aronson FR et al: A randomized phase II trial of continuous infusion (CI) Interleukin-2 (IL-2) or bolus injection (BI) IL-2 plus lymphokine-activated killer cells (LAK) for advanced renal cell carcinoma. Proc Am Soc Clin Oncol 1989 (8):131 (Abstr 509)

37 Calabresi F, Ruggeri EM, Natoli S et al: A phase II trial of adoptive immunotherapy with IL-2 + LAK cells: Preliminary report. 13th Congress of the European Society for Medical Oncology. Lugano (CH) Oct 30 - Nov 1, 1988

38 Kozemy GA, Nicolas JD, Sticklin L et al: Effects of Interleukin-2 immunotherapy on renal function. J Clin Oncol 1988 (6):1170-1176

39 Belldegrun A, Webb DE, Austin AA et al: Effects of Interleukin-2 on renal function in patients receiving immunotherapy for advanced cancer. Am Intern Med 1987 (106):817-822

40 Ettinghausen SE, Puri RK and Rosenberg SA: Increased vascular permeability in organs mediated by the systemic administration of lymphokine-activated killer cells and recombinant interleukin-2 in mice. JNCI 1988 (80):177-188

41 Margolin KA, Rainer AA, Hawkins MJ et al: Interleukin-2 and lymphokine activated killer cell therapy of solid tumors: Analysis of toxicity and management guideline. J Clin Oncol 1989 (7):486-498

42 Belldegrun A, Webb DE, Austin HA et al: Renal toxicity of Interleukin-2 administration in patients with metastatic renal cell cancer: effect of pre-therapy nephrectomy. J Urol 1989 (141):499-503

43 Nora R, Abrams GS and TaitNS: Myocardial toxic effects during recombinant Interleukin-2 therapy. JNCI 1989 (81):59-63

44 Atkins MB, Mier JW, Parkinson DR et al: Hypothyroidism after treatment with Interleukin-2 and lymphokine-activated killer cells. N Engl J Med 1988 (318):1557-1563

45 Gemlo BT, Palladino MA, Jaffe HS et al: Circulating cytokines in patients with metastatic cancer treated with recombinant interleukin-2 and lymphokine-activated killer cells. Cancer Res 1988 (48):5864-5867

46 Giannella G, Pelosi Testa E, Carlini P et al: Fluctuations of plasma B2-microglobulin, soluble interleukin-2 receptor and interferon-gamma concentrations after adoptive immunotherapy with high-dose interleukin-2 and lymphokine-activated killer cells. Immunobiol 1988 (178):305-315

47 Wiebke FA, Rosenberg SA and Lotze MT: Acute immunologic effects of interleukin-2 therapy in cancer patients: decreased delayed type hypersensitivity response and decreased proliferative response to soluble antigens. J Clin Oncol 1988 (6):1440-1449

48 Rosenberg SA, Spiess P and Lafreniere R: A new approach to the adoptive immunotherapy of cancer with tumor infiltrating lymphocytes. Science 1986 (233):1318-1321

49 Spiess PJ, Young JC and Rosenberg SA: In vivo antitumor activity of tumor-infiltrating lymphocytes expanded in recombinant Interleukin-2. JNCI 1987 (79):1067-1075

50 Muul LM, Spiess PJ, Director EP et al: Identification of specific cytolytic immune responses against autologous tumor in humans bearing malignant melanoma. J Immunol 1987 (138):989-995

51 Itoh K, Tilden AB and Balch CM: Interleukin-2 activation of cytotoxic T lymphocytes infiltrating into human metastatic melanomas. Cancer Res 1986 (46):3011-3017

52 Belldegrun A, Munl LM and Rosenberg SA: Interleukin-2 expanded tumor infiltrating lymphocytes human renal cancer: isolation characterization and antitumor activity. Cancer Res 1988 (48):206-214

53 Topalian SL, Muul LM, Salomon D et al: Expansion of human tumor infiltrating lymphocytes for use in immunotherapy trials. J Immunol Methods 1987 (102):127-141

54 Kurnick JJ, Kradin RL, Blumberg R et al: Functional characterization of T lymphocytes propagated from human lung carcinomas. Clin Immunol Immunopathial 1986 (38):367-380

55 Kradin RL, Boyle LA, Preffer FI et al: Tumor-derived interleukin-2 dependent lymphocytes in adoptive immunotherapy of lung cancer. Cancer Immunol Immunother 1987 (24):207-214

56 Rosenberg SA, Packard BS, Aebersold PM et al: Use of tumor infiltrating lymphocytes and Interleukin-2 in the immunotherapy of patients with metastatic melanoma. A preliminary report. N Engl J Med 1988 (319):1676-1680

57 Fisher B, Packard BS, Read EJ et al: Tumor localization of adoptively transferred Indium-111 labeled tumor infiltrating lymphocytes in patients with metastatic melanoma. J Clin Oncol 1989 (7):250-261

58 Kradin RL, Kurnick JJ, Lazarus DS et al: Tumor infiltrating lymphocytes and Interleukin-2 in treatment of advanced cancer. Lancet 1989 (18):577-580

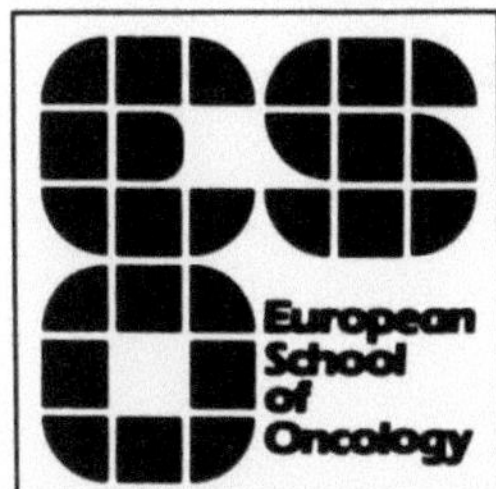

ESO Monographs

Series Editor: U. Veronesi

S. Monfardini, Aviano (Ed.)

The Management of Non-Hodgkin's Lymphomas in Europe

1990. VIII, 92 pp. 13 figs. 12 tabs. Softcover DM 84,–
ISBN 3-540-52297-2

J. C. Holland, New York; **R. Zittoun,** Paris (Eds.)

Psychosocial Aspects of Oncology

1990. VIII, 142 pp. 3 figs. Hardcover DM 82,–
ISBN 3-540-51947-5

A. Breit, Technical University of Munich (Ed.-in-Chief)

Magnetic Resonance in Oncology

A. L. Baert, R. Felix, R. Musumeci, W. Semmler and G. Sze
(Co-Eds.)
1990. XIII, 173 pp. 147 figs. 7 tabs. Hardcover DM 178,–
ISBN 3-540-51054-0

A. B. Miller, Toronto, Ont. (Ed.)

Diet and the Aetiology of Cancer

1989. VII, 73 pp. 2 figs. Hardcover DM 92,–
ISBN 3-540-50681-0

F. Cavalli, Bellinzona (Ed.)

Endocrine Therapy of Breast Cancer III

1989. VII, 65 pp. 26 figs. 7 tabs. Hardcover DM 64,–
ISBN 3-540-50819-8

L. Domellöf, Örebro (Ed.)

Drug Delivery in Cancer Treatment II

Symptom Control, Cytokines, Chemotherapy

1989. VII, 107 pp. 31 figs. Hardcover DM 136,–
ISBN 3-540-51055-9

L. Denis, Antwerpen (Ed.)

The Medical Management of Prostate Cancer

1988. IX, 98 pp. 8 figs. Hardcover DM 82,–
ISBN 3-540-18627-1

B. Winograd, Amsterdam; **M. Peckham,** London;
H. M. Pinedo, Amsterdam (Eds.)

Human Tumour Xenografts in Anticancer Drug Development

1988. XV, 143 pp. 37 figs. Hardcover DM 116,–
ISBN 3-540-18638-7

Also available:

L. Domellöf, Örebro (Ed.)

Drug Delivery in Cancer Treatment

1987. VII, 99 pp. Hardcover DM 82,– ISBN 3-540-18459-7

J. F. Smyth, Edinburgh (Ed.)

Interferons in Oncology

Current Status and Future Directions

1987. VII, 70 pp. Hardcover DM 48,– ISBN 3-540-18019-2

F. Cavalli, Bellinzona (Ed.)

Endocrine Therapy of Breast Cancer

Concepts and Strategies

1986. VII, 120 pp. Hardcover DM 46,– ISBN 3-540-16959-8

A. Goldhirsch, Lugano (Ed.)

Endocrine Therapy of Breast Cancer IV

1990. VIII, 97 pp. 19 figs. 40 tabs. Hardcover DM 68,–
ISBN 3-540-52961-6

E. J. Freireich, University of Texas (Ed.)

New Approaches to the Treatment of Leukaemia

1990. VII, 193 pp. 37 figs. Hardcover DM 148,–
ISBN 3-540-52261-1

L. Tomatis, Lyon (Ed.)

Air Pollution and Human Cancer

1990. VII, 86 pp. 7 figs. 10 tabs. Hardcover DM 78,–
ISBN 3-540-52901-2

L. Domellöf, Örebro (Ed.)

Drug Delivery in Cancer Treatment III

Home Care Symptom Control, Economy, Brain Tumors

1990. VIII, 125 pp. 34 figs. 38 tabs.
Hardcover DM 148,–
ISBN 3-540-52951-9

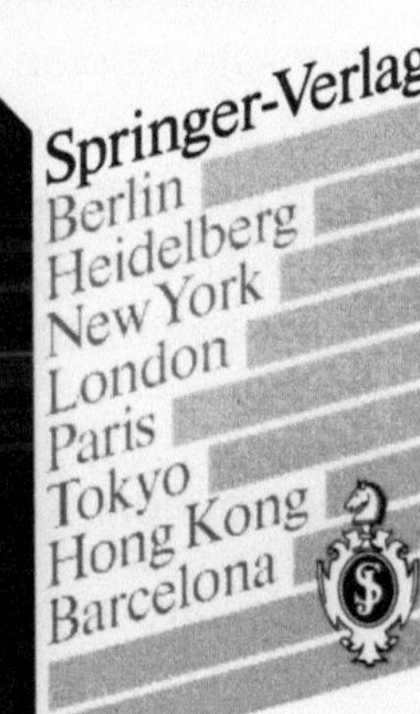

U. Veronesi (Editor-in-Chief); **B. Arnesjø, I. Burn, L. Denis, F. Mazzeo**
(Co-Editors)

Surgical Oncology

A European Handbook

Foreword by I. Burn

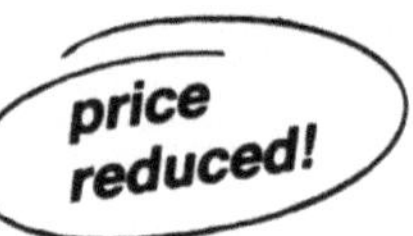

1989. XVIII, 999 pp. 222 figs. 227 tabs. Hardcover DM 198,–
ISBN 3-540-17770-1

…it offers instruction in the fundamental principles which underlie the essentially inter-disciplinary nature of tumor surgery, and provides an excellent survey of the other non-surgical treatment modalities.

The editors of the European Handbook of Surgical Oncology have pursued this design in a consistent fashion. In short, informative, and in most cases readily understandable chapters, the reader is first introduced to the "Biology of Cancer", "Detection and Diagnosis", and the "General Concepts in Cancer Treatment". Particularly worthwhile is the section on "General Concepts in Cancer Treatment", which succeeds in making such interdisciplinary areas as "Radiation Oncology", "Medical Oncology", "Hormones in Cancer Treatment", "Immuno-therapy", as well as the "Psychological Aspects of Surgical Oncology" comprehensible to the oncologic surgeon.

The surgeon is increasingly confronted with surgical emergencies in tumor patients. The section "Emergencies in Cancer Disease", which is devoted to this problem, provides a clear overview of the appropriate emergency surgical procedures. In the section entitled "Rehabili-tation Procedures", various techniques for the operative rehabilitation of tumor patients are described, particularly with respect to the special areas of plastic and orthopedic surgery. It is essential in modern oncologic practice that the therapeutic effects of multidisciplinary treat-ments be evaluated within the framework of controlled clinical trials. This represents the only precise method for assessment of value of various elements within a complex treatment program. "Planning and Evaluation of Cancer Treatment", the section devoted to this problem, contains, among other things, a short but nonetheless clear chapter explaining to the non-statistician the methods commonly used for analysis of recurrence and survival data.

The second half of this comprehensive volume is devoted to organ-specific tumor therapy. Again here, the interdisciplinary treatment possibilities are gone into thoroughly in each chapter…

Annals of Oncology

Distribution rights for Japan: Maruzen Company, Tokyo

Prices are subject to change without notice.

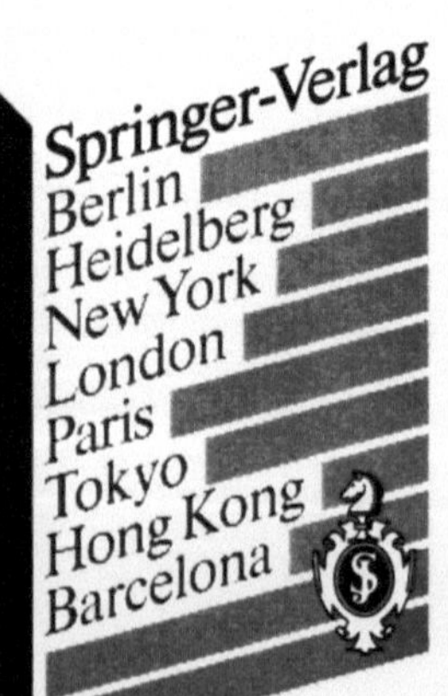

MIX
Papier aus verantwortungsvollen Quellen
Paper from responsible sources
FSC® C105338

If you have any concerns about our products,
you can contact us on
ProductSafety@springernature.com

In case Publisher is established outside the EU,
the EU authorized representative is:
Springer Nature Customer Service Center GmbH
Europaplatz 3, 69115 Heidelberg, Germany

Printed by Libri Plureos GmbH
in Hamburg, Germany